Dependable Delivery Systems Around The Clock!

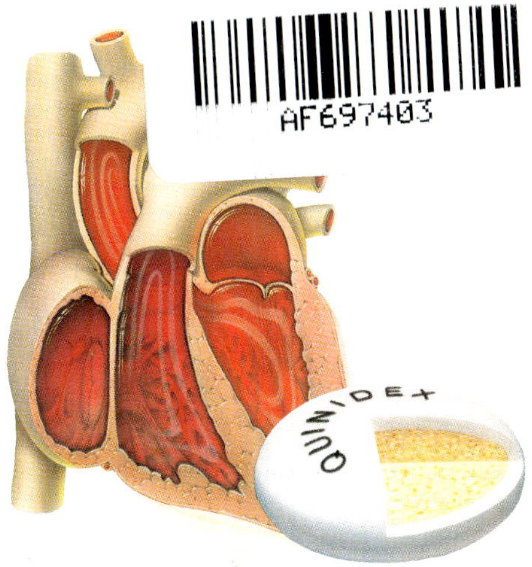

B.I.D.

Twice-a-day dosing* to make life easier for your arrhythmia patients. That's the Quinidex® advantage. Because, like the heart, Quinidex Extentabs® have been uniquely constructed for dependable around-the-clock performance.

**Some patients may require t.i.d. dosing.*

QUINIDEX
EXTENTABS®
(Quinidine Sulfate, USP) 300mg

A·H·ROBINS
Pharmaceutical Division, Richmond, Virginia 23261-6609

Please see prescribing information on the following page.

ECG POCKET GUIDE

ECG POCKET GUIDE

BRADFORD C. LIPMAN, A.B., M.D.
Clinical Instructor in Medicine
Department of Medicine
Division of Cardiology
Emory University School of Medicine
Atlanta, Georgia
Former Fellow in Cardiology
University of Florida School of Medicine
Gainesville, Florida

BERNARD S. LIPMAN, A.B., M.D., F.A.C.C., F.A.C.P., F.C.C.P.
Clinical Professor Emeritus of Medicine (Cardiology)
Emory University School of Medicine
Former Director, Now Consultant, Heart Station
St. Joseph's Hospital
Visiting Physician and Consultant in Cardiology
Grady Memorial Hospital
Consultant in Cardiology
Department of Health and Human Services
Atlanta, Georgia

YEAR BOOK MEDICAL PUBLISHERS, INC.
CHICAGO • LONDON • BOCA RATON

234567890CK91 90 89 88 87

Library of Congress Cataloging-in-Publication Data

Lipman, Bradford C.
ECG pocket guide.

Includes bibliographies and index.
1. Electrocardiography—Handbooks, manuals, etc.
I. Lipman, Bernard S. (Bernard Sylvester), 1920- .
II. Title. [DNLM: 1. Electrocardiography—handbooks.
WG 39 L764e]
RC683.5.E5L55 1987 616.1′207′547 86-26653
ISBN 0-8151-5450-X

Sponsoring Editor: Richard H. Lampert
Manager, Copyediting Services: Frances M. Perveiler
Production Project Manager: Robert Allen Reedtz
Proofroom Supervisor: Shirley E. Taylor

To our family,
To LESLIE JOY, *a devoted mother and understanding wife.*
To LARRY, BOB, *and* BILL, *for their encouragement and love.*

Preface

Yes! Another book on ECG interpretation! Although it has been over 85 years since Einthoven first registered the electrical current from the human heart with his string galvanometer, and although numerous sophisticated diagnostic tools are utilized today, the ECG is still one of the most useful, economical, and available aids in the clinical evaluation of heart disorders.

We have set out to write a simple, basic, concise book with numerous illustrations for the beginner as well as the intermediate ECG interpreter. We attempted to include what we considered essential, important, and commonly seen ECGs. The primary purpose of this book is to give the reader a practical, basic, easily understandable approach for ECG diagnosis "at the bedside."

This "pocket edition" has been written in a format conducive to interpreting the ECG without a lot of complicated, intricate, unnecessary detail. It also serves as a quick reference and review and is bound so that it can be carried in a pocket for ready accessibility. The younger author (B.C.L.), who is also the senior author, is fresh from residency-fellowship post graduate training and is the primary architect for the format. Frequently, the younger author, for the sake of simplicity, eliminated material that the older author attempted to insert with the statement "see reference text." This refers the reader to a more "in depth" discussion in the ECG textbook, the 7th edition of *Clinical Electrocardiography*, co-authored by the older author (B.S.L.). The end result is hopefully an *ECG Pocket Guide* that is accurate yet easily digestible.

Detailed electrophysiologic concepts were omitted, but an attempt was made to include current and commonly accepted basic electrophysiologic theories pertaining to important ECG topics and diagnoses. Refer to the Table of Contents for a list of subjects that we considered essential and pertinent.

Although many of our illustrations are original, we are indebted to Year Book Medical Publishers for permitting us to use some of their illustrations as well as for providing a supplementary source of additional detailed discussions from the reference text *Clinical Electrocardiography*, 7th edition.*

We wish to acknowledge our indebtedness to the many individuals without whose labors, experiments and contributions this book could not have been written. We want to express our deepest gratitude and appreciation to our secretaries and technicians, especially Ms. Betsy DeReus and Ms. Vicki Ostlund for their devoted work; to Armstrong Industries, Northbrook, Illinois, for supplying some of our illustrative rhythms; and to our colleagues and attending staff at Shands Hospital, University of Florida, Gainesville, Florida and St. Joseph's Hospital, Atlanta, Georgia. To the staff of Year Book Medical Publishers we again express our appreciation for their cooperation and counseling which rendered our job immeasurably less difficult.

Most importantly we want to express our gratitude to our family for their patience and encouragement.

BRADFORD C. LIPMAN, M.D.
BERNARD S. LIPMAN, M.D.

---

*Lipman BS, Dunn M, Massie E: *Clinical Electrocardiography*, 7th edition. Chicago, Year Book Medical Publishers, 1984. For detailed references, see bibliography in this reference text.

Introduction

The ECG is a graphic representation of the electrical forces produced by the heart. It is a simple, useful, and practical diagnostic test that has limitations and pitfalls. Knowledge of the clinical data is extremely helpful and important in arriving at an accurate ECG interpretation. There is definitely a distinct advantage of interpreting the ECG immediately "at the bedside."

The ECG interpreter should know that there is a wide range of "normals," and that there may be an overlap between normal and pathologic findings. Coexisting factors such as drugs, electrolytes, body habitus, etc., can influence the ECG tracing. Additionally, technical and "real" pitfalls (myocardial infarction in left bundle branch block, wide QRS complex tachycardias, aberration, preexcitation syndromes [Wolff-Parkinson-White syndrome], etc.) must be recognized to avoid errors in interpretation and treatment. Often, clear-cut diagnoses are not possible. Some tracings may not be unraveled by the most experienced interpreter. The correct ECG diagnosis requires a knowledgeable ECG interpreter with intelligence, judiciousness, proper perspective, and as much clinical data as possible at the time of interpretation.

Contents

1 / Anatomy

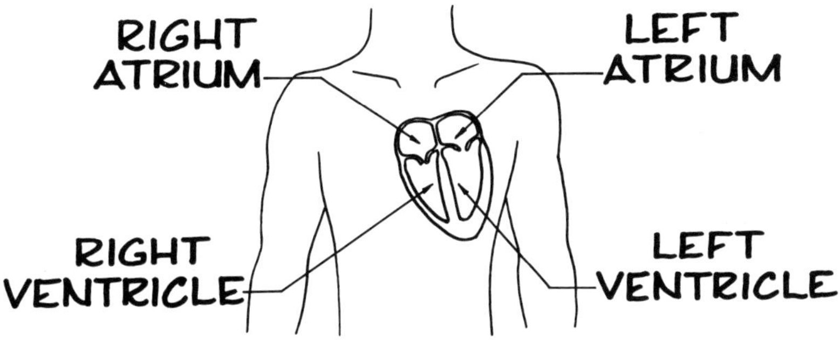

FIG 1–1.
Anatomy of the heart.

A brief review of the heart's anatomy and conducting system is in order. The heart is divided into four chambers: right atrium, right ventricle, left atrium, left ventricle. The upper chambers, right and left atria, receive the blood from the systemic (body) and pulmonary (lung) circulations, respectively. The upper chambers are *thin-walled* and propel blood to the right and left ventricles, respectively. The lower right and left ventricles are *thick-walled* chambers that constitute the majority of the heart's mass or weight. The right ventricle pumps blood into the lungs (pulmonary circulation); the left ventricle pumps blood into the body (systemic circulation).

Normally, the amount of blood that enters the right atrium is the same amount that enters the left atrium. Both atria contract (atrial kick) to propel blood into their respective ventricles. The right and left ventricles then contract together to pump blood into the pulmonary and systemic circulations. A normal heart beat consists of contraction of both atria followed by contraction of both ventricles. This orderly process of contraction is initiated and maintained by the heart's electrical forces, which are recorded by the electrocardiogram or *ECG*.

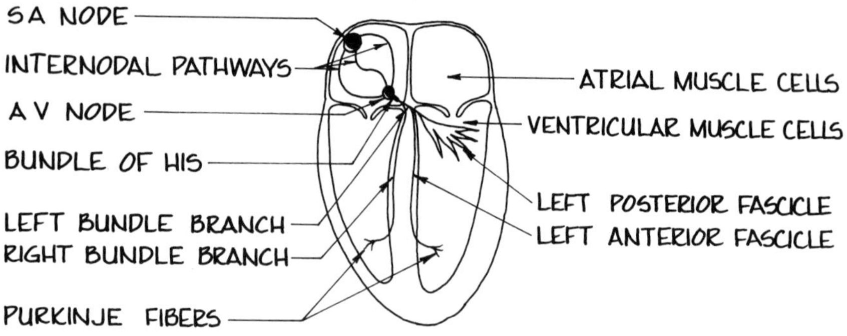

FIG 1–2.
Impulse formation and specialized conducting system of the heart. Normally, the initiating pacemaker cells are located in the *SA* (sinoatrial) node. Impulses are conducted through the specialized conducting system shown above at a very rapid rate. The deflections in the ECG represent excitation only in the atrial and ventricular muscle cells.

IMPULSE FORMATION AND CONDUCTION

The *ECG* is simply a display of the electrical currents that are generated by the heart and are spread through the surrounding tissue to the surface of the body. The electrical impulses are picked up by the surface electrodes and are then recorded in the ECG.

Involved in the process of electrical impulse formation, conduction, and mechanical contraction are three types of heart cells:

1. *Pacemaker cells* initiate the electrical impulses. Normally, pacemaker cells in the sinoatrial (SA) node start the electrical sequence; however, other pacemaker cells are located throughout the heart.
2. *Specialized conducting cells* conduct the electrical impulses. The specialized conducting system consists of the SA node, atrial internodal pathways, atrioventricular (AV) node, bundle of His, right and left bundle branches, left anterior and posterior fascicles, and Purkinje fibers.
3. *Muscle cells* have the functions of electrical conduction *and* mechanical contraction; these cells make up the majority of the mass of the atria and ventricles.

The pacemaker cells and specialized conducting cells transmit impulses too rapidly to be recorded in the ECG. *Importantly, the surface ECG records electrical activity from only the muscle cells.* Stimulation of muscle cells causes mechanical contraction, which produces the normal heartbeat.

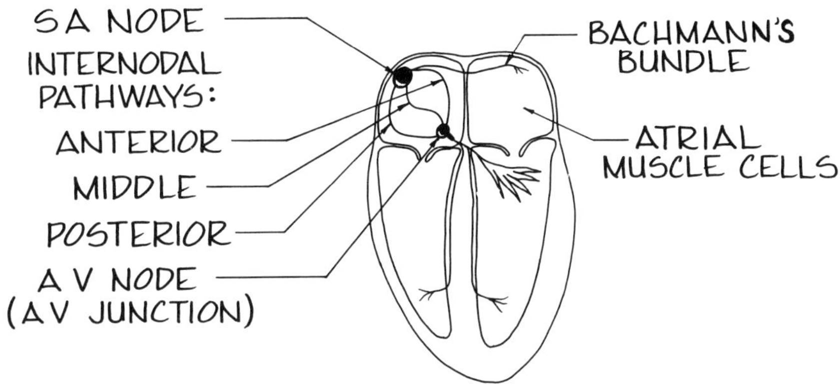

FIG 1–3.
Atrial conducting system. *SA* (sinoatrial) node, internodal pathways (anterior, middle, posterior), Bachmann's bundle, *AV* (atrioventricular) node (AV junction). When the atrial muscle cells are activated, they conduct more slowly and produce the P wave in the ECG.

ATRIAL CONDUCTING SYSTEM

The electrical impulses normally originate in the SA node. This is the primary pacemaker of the heart and is located in the upper part of the right atrium. The impulses, on their way to the AV node, travel through three main internodal conduction pathways in and around both atria (anterior, middle, and posterior internodal pathways) and in a pathway called Bachmann's bundle leading to the left atrium.

Stimulation of the slower-conducting muscle cells of both atria produces the P wave in the ECG. *The P wave represents electrical excitation of the atrial muscle cells.* This electrical stimulation is followed by mechanical contraction of the atria.

Electrical impulses in the atria converge low in the right atrium where they enter the AV node (also called AV junction). The AV node acts as a way station, a "delay area," where impulses from both atria are slowed down. This delay gives time for the atria to contract and propel ("kick") their contents into their respective ventricles.

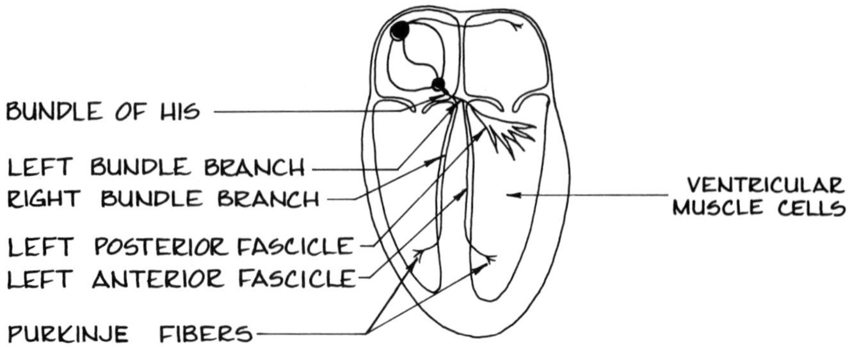

FIG 1–4.
Ventricular conducting system. Bundle of His, RBB, LBB, left anterior fascicle, left posterior fascicle, Purkinje fibers. When the ventricular muscle cells are activated, they conduct more slowly and produce the QRS complex in the ECG.

VENTRICULAR CONDUCTING SYSTEM

After the brief delay in the AV node, the impulses proceed down a specialized conducting pathway called the bundle of His. The bundle of His quickly divides into two pathways: right bundle branch (RBB), which traverses the right ventricle, and left bundle branch (LBB), which traverses the left ventricle.

The short main LBB further divides into anterior and posterior fascicles, which supply the anterior-superior and posterior-inferior regions of the left ventricle, respectively. Both RBB and LBB divide into smaller branches and finally into the terminal conducting system in the ventricles called Purkinje cells. From the Purkinje cells, the muscle cells of both ventricles are stimulated, which produces the QRS complex in the ECG. *The QRS complex represents electrical excitation of the ventricular muscle cells.* This electrical excitation of the muscle cells is followed by mechanical contraction of the ventricles.

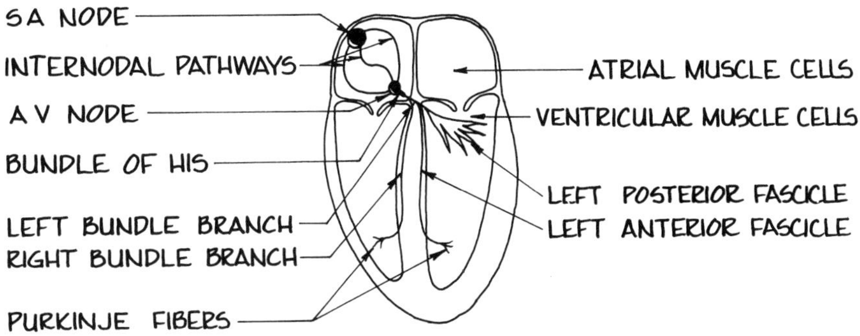

FIG 1–5.
Normal sequence of electrical activation in the heart. *SA,* sinoatrial; *AV,* atrioventricular.

SEQUENCE OF HEART ACTIVATION

The normal sequence of electrical activation in the heart is as follows:

SA node
↓
Internodal pathways and Bachmann's bundle
↓
Muscle cells of both atria (producing the P wave)
↓
AV node
↓
Bundle of His
↙ ↘
Right bundle branch — Left bundle branch
Left bundle branch ↙ ↘
Left anterior fascicle — Left posterior fascicle
Right bundle branch, Left anterior fascicle, Left posterior fascicle
↓
Purkinje cells
↓
Muscle cells of both ventricles
(producing the QRS complex)

2 / ECG Leads

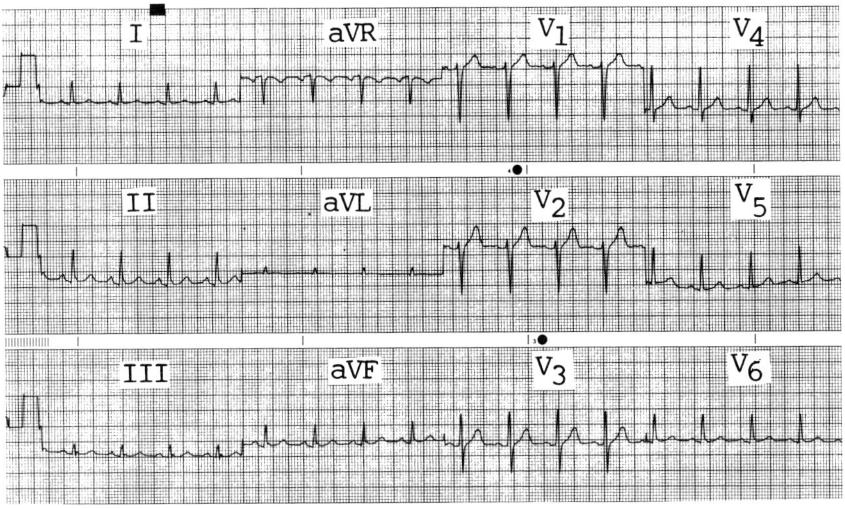

FIG 2–1.
Normal 12-lead ECG. Three leads are recorded simultaneously using a three-channel machine.

The conventional ECG records 12 leads. These twelve leads consist of the following:

1. Six *limb or extremity leads* designated standard limb leads I, II, III, and unipolar limb leads aVR, aVL, aVF. These leads are derived from *electrodes* placed on the right arm, left arm, and left leg. The right leg electrode acts as a grounding electrode.
2. Six *chest or precordial leads* designated V_1, V_2, V_3, V_4, V_5, V_6. These leads are derived from six *electrodes* placed on the chest in designated areas.

The conventional ECG machine records one lead at a time. Other machines may record 3 leads, 6 leads, or 12 leads simultaneously.

ELECTRODE PLACEMENT

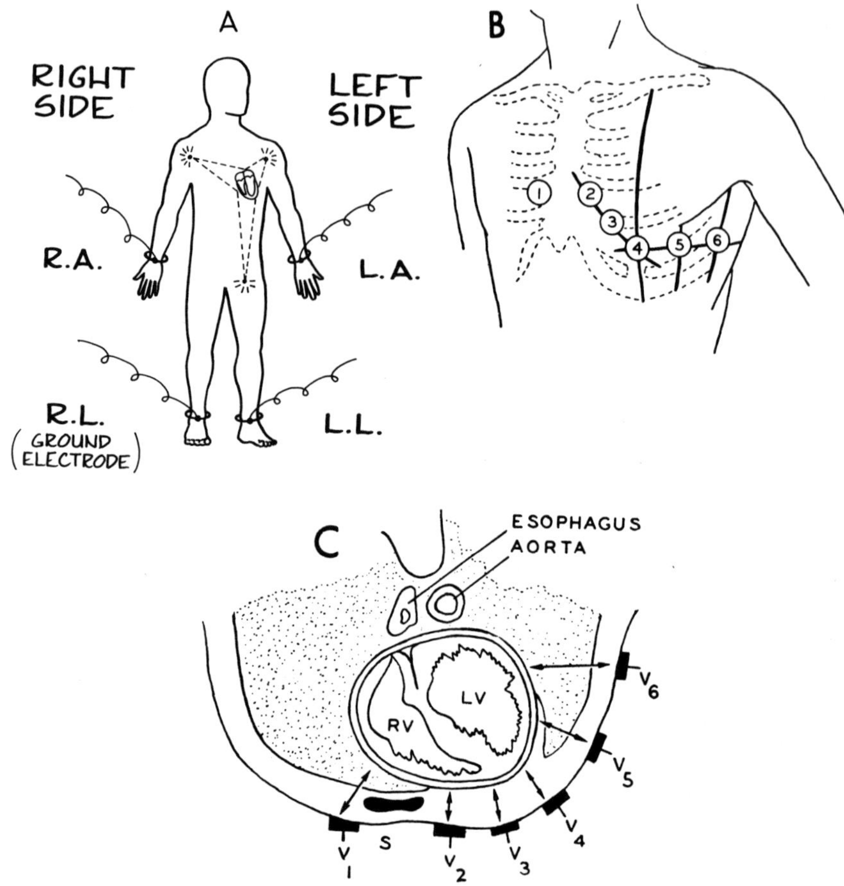

FIG 2–2.
Electrode placement sites. **A,** limb electrode sites. **B,** chest electrode sites (leads V_1 to V_6) in the frontal view. **C,** chest electrode sites (leads V_1 to V_6) in the cross-sectional view. *RA,* right arm; *LA,* left arm; *RL,* right leg; *LL,* left leg; *RV,* right ventricle; *LV,* left ventricle.

ELECTRODE PLACEMENT

Placement of the *limb* electrodes is shown (Fig 2–2,*A*). Electrodes are placed on the right arm (RA), left arm (LA), and left leg (LL). The right leg (RL) electrode is a ground electrode. The electrode on each extremity records electrical forces from the heart as viewed from the junction of that extremity with the body. In other words, the right and left arm electrodes record forces presented to the right and left shoulders, respectively; the left leg electrode records forces presented to the left thigh. As an example, a patient with a left thigh amputation may have the electrode placed above the amputation site without altering the ECG.

The illustrations on the right (Fig 2–2,*B*,*C*) show positions of the *chest* electrodes in both frontal and cross-sectional views. The conventional six chest electrode sites are as follows:

V_1: fourth intercostal space, right sternal border
V_2: fourth intercostal space, left sternal border
V_3: midway between V_2 and V_4
V_4: fifth or sixth interspace (where apex of the heart is felt), midclavicular line
V_5: anterior axillary line, same level with V_4
V_6: midaxillary line, same level with V_4 and V_5

Note the positions of the chest electrode sites in the cross-sectional view (Fig 2–2, C). Electrodes V_1 and V_2 overlie the right ventricle; electrodes V_4, V_5, and V_6 overlie the left ventricle. Electrode V_3 overlies the interventricular septum.

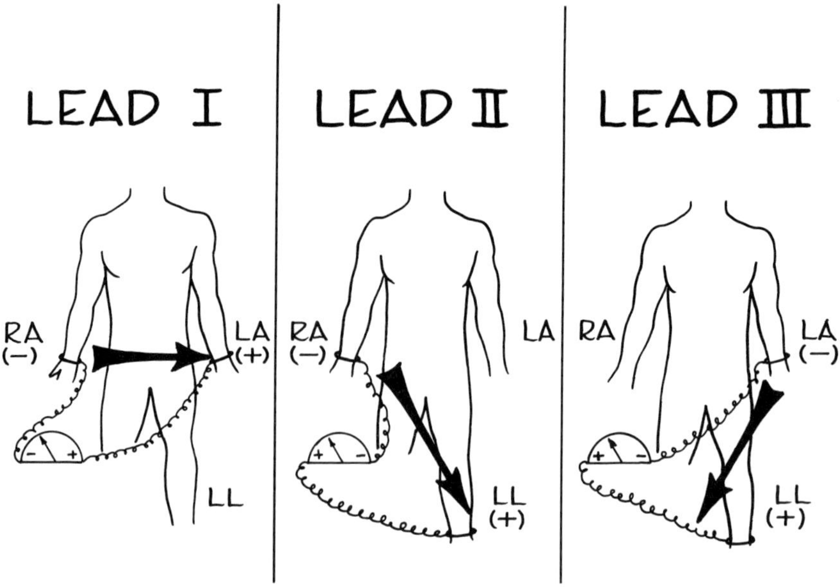

FIG 2–3.
Electrode sites used to determine the three standard limb leads. Arbitrarily, in *lead I,* the left arm is positive; in *leads II* and *III,* the left leg is positive. The *arrow* points toward the positive end of each standard limb lead. *RA,* right arm; *LA,* left arm; *LL,* left leg.

STANDARD LIMB LEADS

The six limb leads are divided into three bipolar and three unipolar leads. The *bipolar* leads are designated *standard* leads I, II, III. Each *bipolar* lead is actually a tracing of the electrical forces recorded between two extremities at one time. The *unipolar* leads record electrical forces from one extremity at a time in relation to a central terminal. The illustrations show the three *bipolar standard limb leads* (I, II, III) and the two *limb electrodes* that are used to record each bipolar lead:

Lead I: right arm to left arm
Lead II: right arm to left leg
Lead III: left arm to left leg

Each bipolar lead (I, II, or III) has a designated positive (+) and negative (−) end that should be remembered. Arbitrarily, the left arm is positive in lead I, and the left leg is positive in leads II and III.

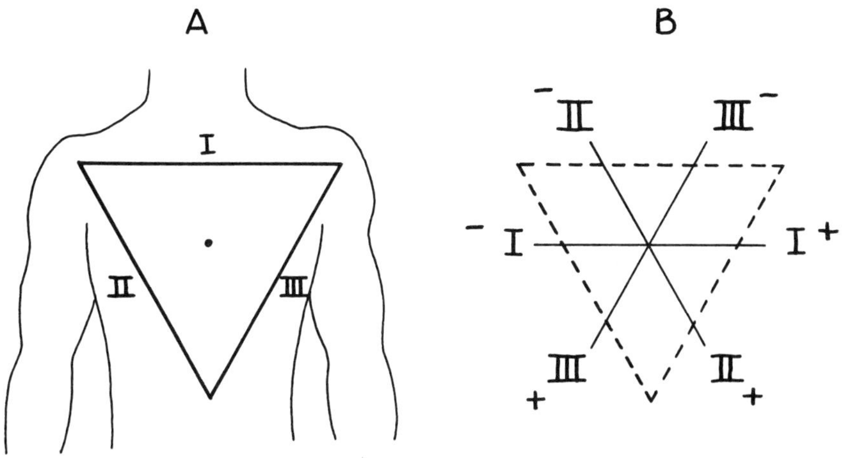

FIG 2–4.
A, the equilateral triangle of Einthoven formed by standard limb leads *I, II,* and *III.* **B,** the triaxial reference system formed by transposing the three sides of the Einthoven triangle onto a central point. Note the positive and negative ends of the three standard limb leads.

EINTHOVEN TRIANGLE

The three standard leads (I, II, III) may be transposed into an equilateral triangle called the Einthoven triangle. The Einthoven triangle concept postulates that the three limb leads form an equilateral triangle with the heart in the center of the triangle (Fig 2–4,*A*).

When the three sides of the triangle are transposed to a common central point, a *triaxial* (three axis) *reference system* is produced (Fig 2–4,*B*). This reference system is useful in determining axis, which will be discussed in chapter 4.

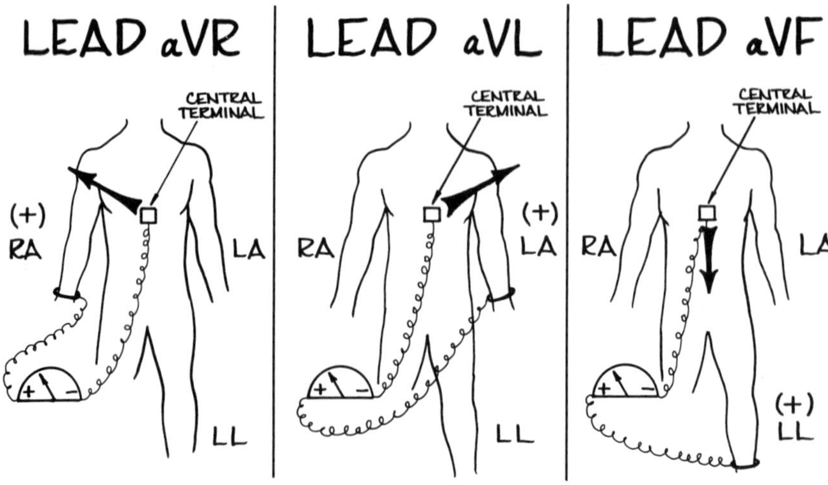

FIG 2–5.
Electrode sites used to determine the three unipolar limb leads. Note that the unipolar technique utilizes a central terminal as a reference point. In *aVR,* the right arm is positive; in *aVL,* the left arm is positive; in *aVF,* the left leg is positive. The *arrow* points toward the positive end of each unipolar limb lead. *RA,* right arm; *LA,* left arm; *LL,* left leg.

UNIPOLAR LIMB LEADS

The three unipolar limb leads are aVR, aVL, and aVF.* Each lead is *unipolar* as opposed to *bipolar,* because each specific lead represents the heart's electrical forces recorded solely from that specific limb electrode. The unipolar technique utilizes a central terminal as a *negative* reference point and the specific limb electrode as the *positive* recording electrode. (See reference text regarding the formation of the central terminal.)

The above figures show the three *unipolar limb leads* (aVR, aVL, aVF) and the specific *limb electrodes* that record the heart's electrical activity utilizing the central terminal as a reference point:

Lead aVR: central terminal to right arm

Lead aVL: central terminal to left arm

Lead aVF: central terminal to left leg (or left *foot*)

Each unipolar lead (aVR, aVL, aVF) has a designated positive (+) and negative (−) end that should be remembered. Arbitrarily, the right arm is positive in aVR, the left arm is positive in aVL, and the left leg is positive in aVF.

*"a" stands for augmented; "V" refers to unipolar; "R" stands for right arm; "L" stands for left arm; "F" refers to left leg.

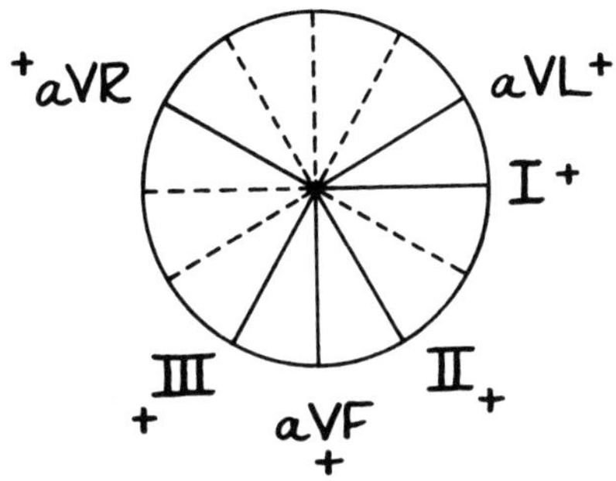

FIG 2–6.
The hexaxial reference system is formed by adding the unipolar limb leads *(aVR, aVL, aVF)* to the triaxial reference system (see p. 11). Note that the designated positive ends of the six limb leads are *solid lines,* and the negative ends are *dashed lines.*

HEXAXIAL REFERENCE SYSTEM

The three unipolar leads may be transposed onto the *triaxial reference system* (see p. 11) to form a *hexaxial (six axes) reference system.* The figure shows the six limb leads (three standard and three unipolar) in the hexaxial reference system with their designated positive ends. This system is very important in determining the axis or major direction of the heart's electrical forces when viewed from the front of the body (frontal plane) (see chapter 4).

CHEST LEADS

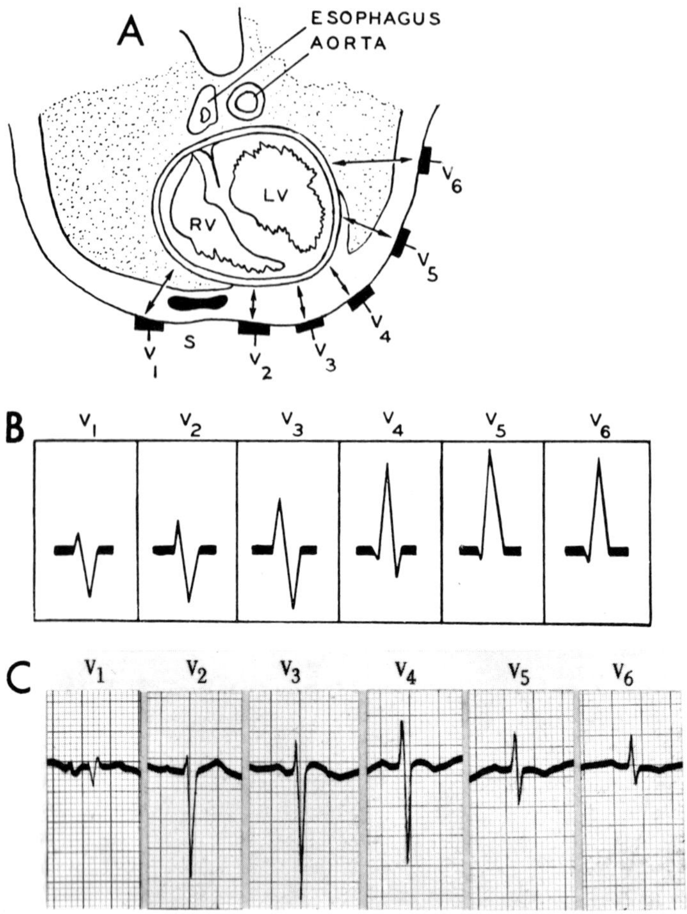

FIG 2–7.
A, placement of the chest electrodes in the cross-sectional view. Normally, electrodes V_1 and V_2 overlie the right ventricle; electrode V_3 overlies the interventricular septum; and electrodes V_4, V_5, V_6 overlie the left ventricle. **B,** normal R wave progression in the chest leads. The transition zone occurs in lead V_3. **C,** poor R wave progression. The transition zone occurs later in the lead V_5.

CHEST LEADS

R Wave Progression

Each chest electrode records in a *unipolar* fashion. In other words, each chest electrode records the heart's electrical forces in reference to a central terminal. The conventional chest leads are designated V_1, V_2, V_3, V_4, V_5, V_6. It is important that the six chest electrodes are placed in their correct positions (see Fig 2–2,*B*).

The left ventricle is the larger of the two ventricles and lies to the left and behind the right ventricle (see Fig 2–7,*A*). The chest electrodes, when placed in their proper positions, record depolarization of the ventricles (QRS complexes) that become progressively more positive from lead V_1 to lead V_6 (Fig 2–7,*B*). The gradual increase in the positive QRS deflections from lead V_1 to V_6 is known as *R wave progression.* Normally, the *transition zone* where the predominantly negative QRS deflections (leads V_1 and V_2) become predominantly positive deflections (R wave becomes greater than S wave) occurs in leads V_3 or V_4.

The concept of *"poor R wave progression"* signifies that the QRS deflections are predominantly negative in leads V_1 to V_4 and positive in V_5 or V_6. The transition zone occurs late in leads V_5 or V_6 (Fig 2–7,*C*).

Poor R wave progression is abnormal and may be seen in the following:

1. Anterior myocardial infarction
2. Left bundle branch block (LBBB)
3. Left ventricular hypertrophy
4. Chronic obstructive pulmonary disease (COPD)

3 / Basic ECG Principles

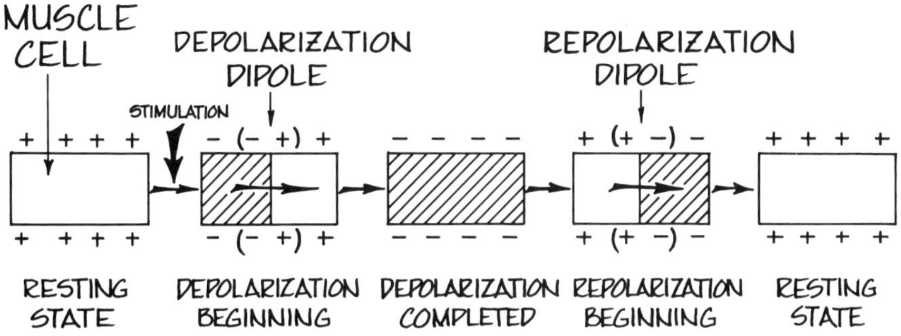

FIG 3–1.
Depolarization and repolarization in a single muscle cell. The *hatched lines* represent depolarization of the muscle cell. During *depolarization,* the positive surface charges change to negative surface charges. Dipoles are pairs of electrical charges. *The depolarization dipoles consist of a positive charge followed by a negative charge* so that the positive charge leads the activation wave. During *repolarization,* the negative surface charges change to positive surface charges. *The repolarization dipoles consist of a negative charge followed by a positive charge.* When repolarization is completed, the myocardial cells return to their resting electrical state.

DEPOLARIZATION AND REPOLARIZATION

Each heartbeat is comprised of two electrical processes: *depolarization* and *repolarization.* During *depolarization,* the positive electrical charges on the surface of the myocardial cells change to negative charges. The muscle cells are activated to contract during depolarization.

Depolarization is followed by *repolarization,* return to the resting electrical state. During repolarization, the negative surface charges return to positive surface charges. Repolarization or "recharging" is necessary before depolarization can recur. If the myocardial cells are not allowed to repolarize fully (return to their resting electrical state), the cells will be *refractory* to the next electrical impulse. In other words, the depolarized cells are unable to be stimulated to contract again until they are repolarized.

Thus, every depolarization (electrical activation) is followed by repolarization (return to the resting electrical state). Myocardial cells are refractory to further impulses until repolarization has been completed or nearly completed.

RECORDING DEPOLARIZATION AND REPOLARIZATION

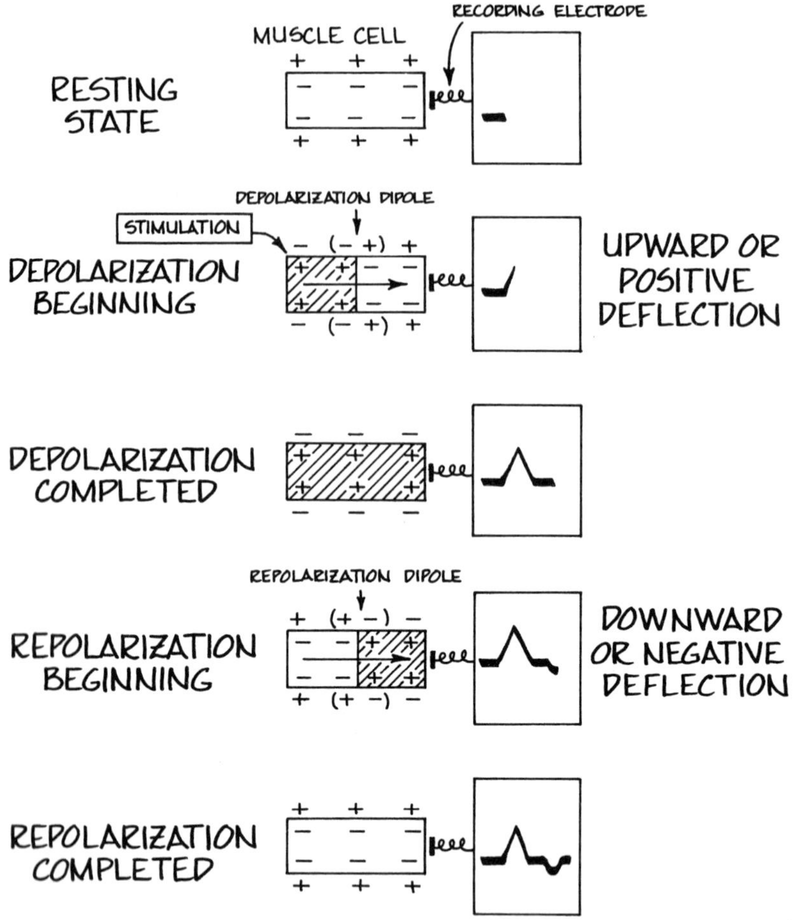

FIG 3–2.
The recorded deflections of depolarization and repolarization when a muscle cell is stimulated. An upward deflection is recorded when the electrode faces the positive side of the depolarization dipole. A downward deflection is recorded when the electrode faces the negative side of the repolarization dipole.

RECORDING DEPOLARIZATION AND REPOLARIZATION

The ECG records the electrical processes of depolarization and repolarization for each heartbeat. Figure 3–2 illustrates an electrode recording depolarization and repolarization in a single muscle cell. Upon electrical stimulation, depolarization is represented by a dipole (pair of electrical charges) consisting of a *positive* (+) charge followed by a *negative* (−) charge. Repolarization is represented by a dipole with a *negative* (−) charge followed by a *positive* (+) charge.

An electrode that faces the positive side of the *depolarization* dipole records an upright or positive deflection. When depolarization or electrical activation is completed, repolarization or return to the resting electrical state follows. The same electrode, this time facing the negative side of the *repolarization* dipole, records a downward or negative deflection.

Depolarization (electrical stimulation) cannot occur until repolarization (return to the resting state) is completed. Both electrical processes occur in the atria and in the ventricles and are recorded in the ECG.

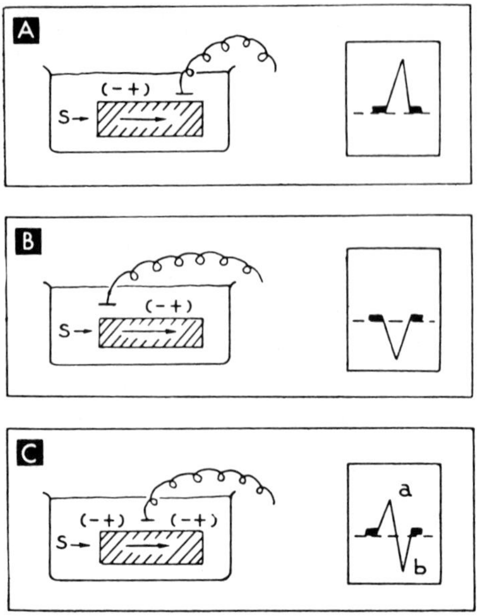

FIG 3–3.
Electrode records upward (positive) or downward (negative) deflection depending on the location of the electrode and the direction of the depolarization dipole.

CONTOUR OF ECG DEFLECTIONS

The direction, size, and shape of the ECG deflections recorded by an electrode are determined by a number of factors such as the site of the electrode, the distance between the electrode and muscle cells, thickness of the chest wall, electrolyte abnormalities, intrinsic cardiac disease, etc. However, two major factors that determine the contour of the ECG deflection include (1) the location of the electrode on the body and (2) the direction of the cardiac impulses or dipoles in relation to the position of the electrode.

In Figure 3–3, note that if the direction of the depolarization impulse is moving toward the electrode, a positive or upward deflection will be recorded (Fig 3–3,*A*, electrode faces positive side of dipole). Conversely, as the depolarization impulse travels away from the recording electrode, a negative or downward deflection will be recorded (Fig 3–3,*B*, electrode faces negative side of dipole). In Figure 3–3,*C*, the electrode initially faces the positive side of the depolarization dipole and records a positive deflection; but, as the dipole passes under and then away from the electrode, a negative deflection is recorded.

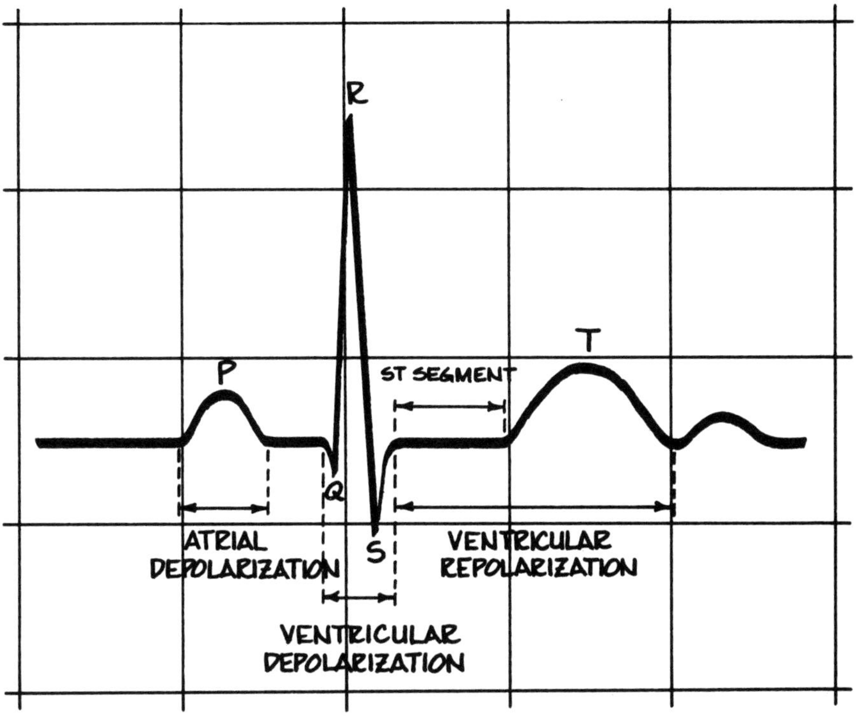

FIG 3–4.
The *P* wave represents atrial depolarization; the QRS complex represents ventricular depolarization. The *ST* segment and *T* wave depict ventricular repolarization. Atrial repolarization is buried in the QRS complex.

DEPOLARIZATION AND REPOLARIZATION DEFLECTIONS IN THE ECG

The depolarization and repolarization processes are recorded as deflections in the ECG for both the atria and the ventricles. *The P wave represents depolarization of the atria. The QRS complex represents depolarization of the ventricles.* The QRS complex is much larger than the P wave, because the ventricles are larger and comprise more muscle mass than the atria.

Repolarization of the ventricles is represented by the ST segment and T wave. Repolarization of the atria occurs at about the same time as depolarization of the ventricles. The deflection produced by atrial repolarization is small and is usually buried in the QRS complex.

The normal electrical excitation of the heart recorded in the ECG consists of a P wave (atrial beat) followed by a QRS complex, ST segment, and T wave (ventricular beat).

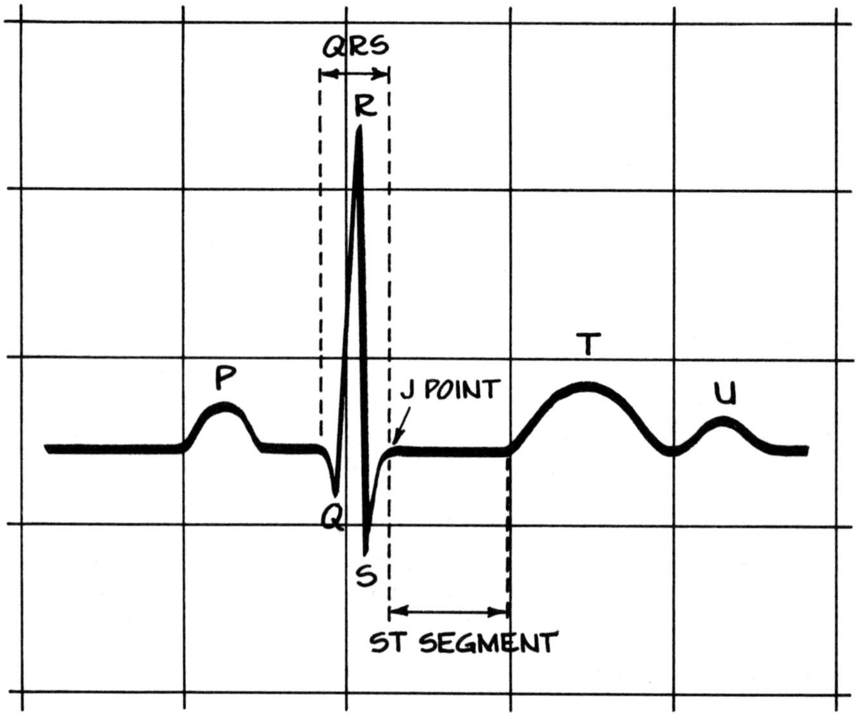

FIG 3–5.
Normal ECG deflections.

ECG NOMENCLATURE

Nomenclature of the deflections and waves in the normal ECG include the following:

P wave: depolarization of right and left atria.

QRS complex: depolarization of right and left ventricles.

ST segment: beginning of ventricular repolarization measured from the end of the QRS complex to the beginning of the T wave. The beginning of the ST segment is termed *J point.*

T wave: repolarization of right and left ventricles.

U wave: not always seen, but when present, it immediately follows the T wave and probably represents late repolarization.

Two important points to note are as follows:

1. The ventricles contain the majority of the heart muscle or mass (left ventricle much more than right ventricle), and this is the reason the QRS complex is much larger than the P wave.
2. The deflection representing repolarization of the atria is small and is usually buried in the much larger QRS complex.

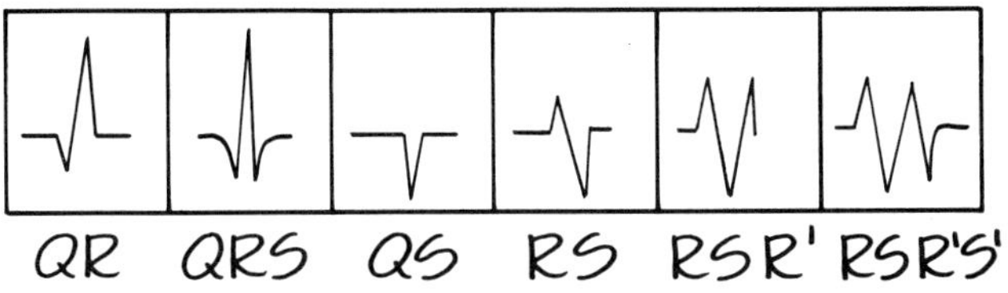

FIG 3–6.
The various configurations of the QRS complex.

TERMINOLOGY OF QRS CONFIGURATIONS

Ventricular depolarization produces the QRS complex, which can have various configurations. The terminology of deflections in a QRS complex is as follows (see figure):

Q wave: initial downward deflection
R wave: first upward deflection
S wave: initial downward deflection following the R wave
R′ wave: second upward deflection following the S wave
S′ wave: second downward deflection following the R wave
QS wave: entire QRS complex consists of a negative deflection

A capital or large letter (Q,R,S) denotes a large deflection. Usually a noncapitalized or small letter (q,r,s) denotes a small deflection.

ECG MEASUREMENTS

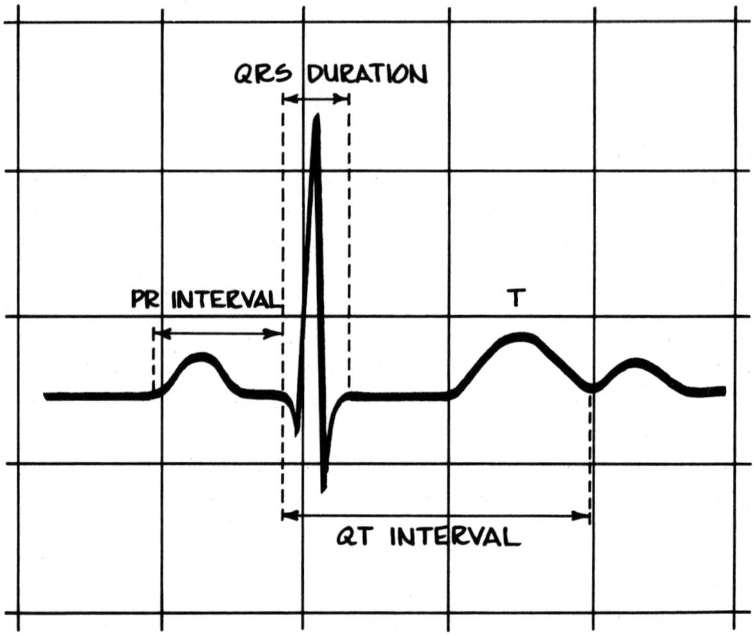

FIG 3–7.
Normal ECG measurements.

ECG MEASUREMENTS

Basic ECG measurements (Fig 3–7) include the following:

1. *P-R interval:* interval measured from the beginning of P wave to the beginning of the QRS complex. This interval represents the time for the impulse to travel from the SA node through the specialized atrial conduction pathways, entire musculature of both atria, AV node, Bundle of His, and the ventricular bundle branches to the Purkinje cells in the ventricles. Note that the P-R interval includes depolarization of atrial muscle cells (P wave) and passage of the impulse to the point of ventricular muscle stimulation.

2. *QRS duration:* interval from the beginning to the end of the QRS complex. This interval represents depolarization of both ventricles.

3. *Q-T interval:* interval measured from the beginning of QRS complex to the end of the T wave. This varies inversely with the heart rate, and is termed Q-T_c when the Q-T interval is *corrected* for the heart rate. See Table 1 for normal Q-T values corrected for heart rate. If the Q-T interval is prolonged, fatal arrhythmias may arise.

Normal time intervals in the adult include the following:

P-R interval: 0.12–0.20 second
QRS duration: 0.06–0.10 second
Q-T interval: varies inversely with heart rate (see Table 1)

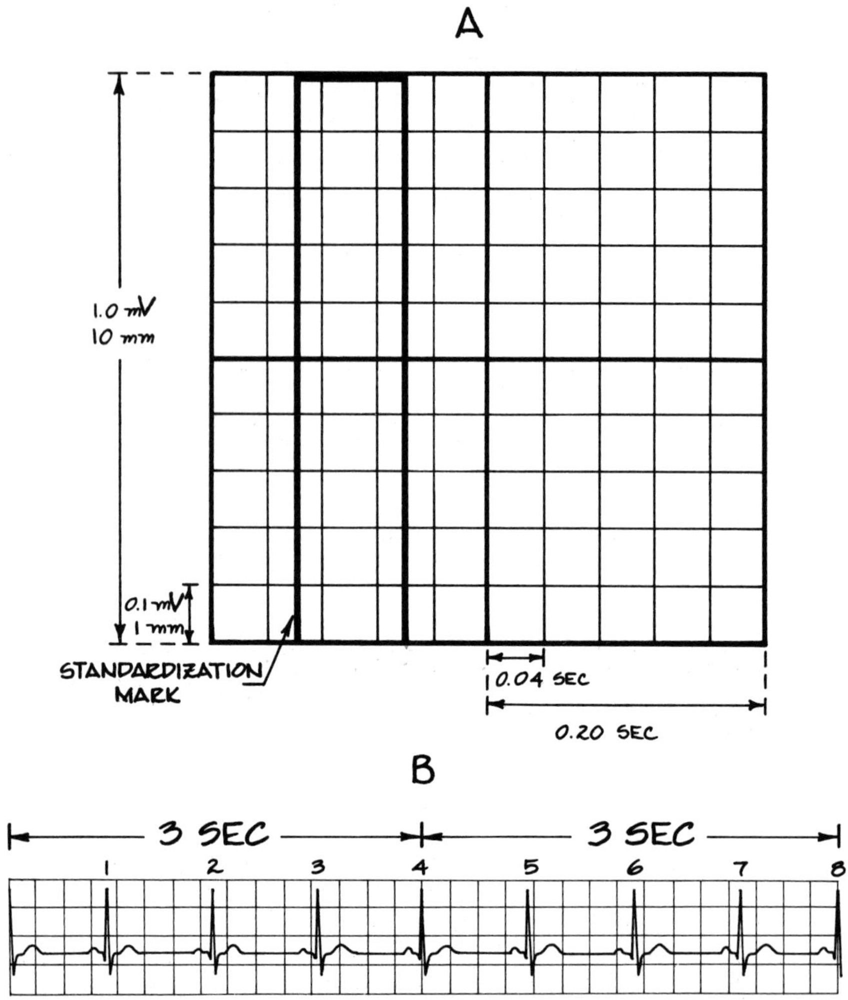

FIG 3–8.
A, enlarged diagrammatic illustration of ECG paper. Normal standardization is 10-mm height (*ten small boxes*) in the vertical direction (1.0 mV). Each small box equals *1 mm* or *0.1 mV*. Standard recording speed is 25 mm/sec. At this speed, each small box in the horizontal direction equals *0.04* second; *five small boxes* (one large square) equal *0.20* second. **B,** heart rate can be calculated by counting the number of QRS complexes within two 3-second markers (6 seconds) and multiplying by ten. In this example, there are eight QRS complexes within a 6-second interval. The heart rate is 10 × 8, which equals 80 beats/min.

HEART RATE DETERMINATION I

Heart rate can be readily determined from the ECG. The standard recording speed of the ECG paper is 25 mm/sec. At this speed, each small box in the horizontal direction equals 0.04 second. A large box consists of five small squares, and equals 0.20 second. The vertical direction in the ECG measures voltage. When the ECG is standardized to the conventional 10 mm of height (Fig 3–8,*A*), each small box equals 0.1 mV, 1 mm of height.

Heart rate is calculated as the number of heart beats per minute (beats/min). In the ECG, heart rate can be determined by counting the number of P waves (atrial rate) or QRS complexes (ventricular rate) in a specified time period. One easy method involves counting the number of QRS complexes in a 6-second period and multiplying that number by ten. This gives the number of heartbeats (heart rate) in 60 seconds. Six seconds in a standard ECG comprises 30 large boxes (30 times 0.20 second per large square equals 6 seconds). Most ECGs have small vertical hatched lines in the margins, which represent 3-second intervals. Simply count the number of QRS complexes in two of these 3-second intervals (6 seconds) and multiply by ten to determine the heart rate per minute (Fig 3–8,*B*).

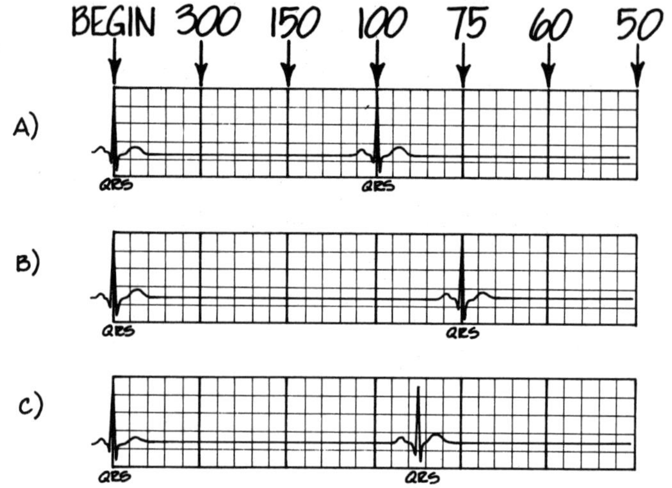

FIG 3–9.
Determination of heart rate. **A,** counting from initial R wave to next R wave *(three large squares),* heart rate is 100 beats/min. **B,** counting from initial R wave to next R wave *(four large squares),* heart rate is 75 beats/min. *C,* counting from initial R wave to next R wave *(3½ large squares),* a heart rate between 75 and 100 beats/min must be estimated: 87 beats/min is appropriate.

HEART RATE DETERMINATION II

Another rapid method for determining heart rate involves memorizing the sequence of numbers shown above (300, 150, 100, 75, 60, 50). Note that each number corresponds to a heavy black line, one *large square* (0.20-second interval). The interval between two successive P waves, *P-P interval,* determines atrial rate; the interval between two successive R waves, *R-R interval,* determines ventricular rate. In normal sinus rhythm, the P wave and QRS complex track together, and the heart rate calculated by using either the P-P interval or R-R interval will be the same.

Using the distance between two successive QRS complexes (R-R interval) to calculate the heart rate, find an R wave superimposed on a heavy black line. Beginning at this point, count the number of heavy black lines or *large squares* to the next R wave. Using the "now-memorized" sequence of numbers, heart rate is determined by the distance between the two successive R waves measured by the *large squares.*

The heart rate numbers are derived by dividing the specific number of successive large squares into 300. For example, if the interval from one R wave to the next R wave is *one* large square, the heart rate is 300 beats/min. If the interval is *two* large squares, the heart rate is 150 beats/min. If the interval is *three* large squares, the heart rate is 100 beats/min, etc. For heart rates slower than 50 beats/min, the next "heart rate" numbers to remember (which coincide with the heavy black lines) are 43, 37, 33, and 30 (see Table 2).

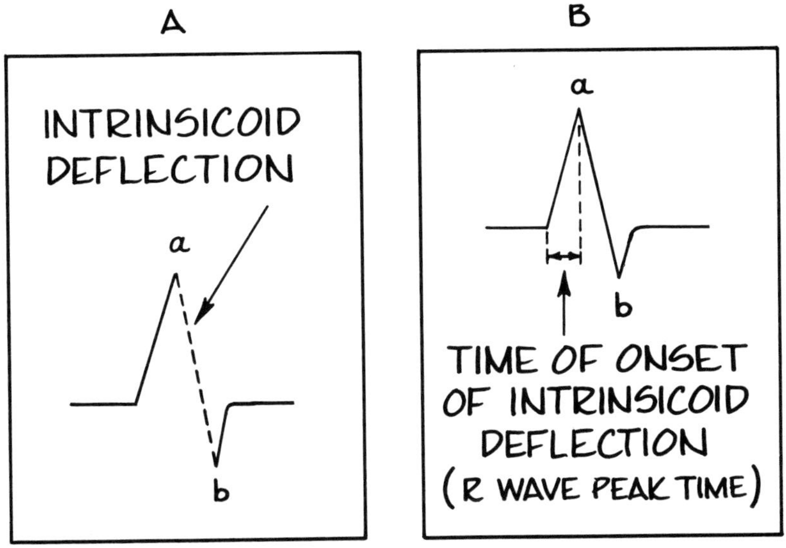

FIG 3–10.
A, intrinsicoid deflection represented by line *ab.* It is the downward deflection after the peak of the R wave. **B,** the *time of onset of intrinsicoid deflection* (R wave peak time) represented by the distance from the beginning of the QRS complex to the peak of the R wave.

INTRINSICOID DEFLECTION

Intrinsicoid deflection is an important concept useful in diagnosing bundle branch blocks (see chapter 6) and ventricular hypertrophy (see chapter 8). The intrinsicoid deflection represents the instant when the depolarization impulse in the ventricles reaches the site under the recording electrode. In the QRS complex, the R wave (initial positive deflection) represents the depolarization impulse approaching the area beneath the electrode. When the impulse reaches the area under the electrode, the R wave is at its peak. As the impulse moves away from the electrode, a downward deflection is recorded. This downward deflection is called the *intrinsicoid deflection* (Fig 3–10,*A*).

The *time of onset of the intrinsicoid deflection,* also referred to as the *R wave peak time* (Fig 3–10,*B*), is measured from the beginning of the QRS complex to the peak of the R wave (or R′ if present). In the presence of bundle branch block or ventricular hypertrophy, the depolarization impulse takes a longer-than-normal period of time to reach the recording electrode. The longer period of time delays the onset of the intrinsicoid deflection. Prolongation of the time of onset of the intrinsicoid deflection is an important criterion for diagnosing ventricular hypertrophy and bundle branch block.

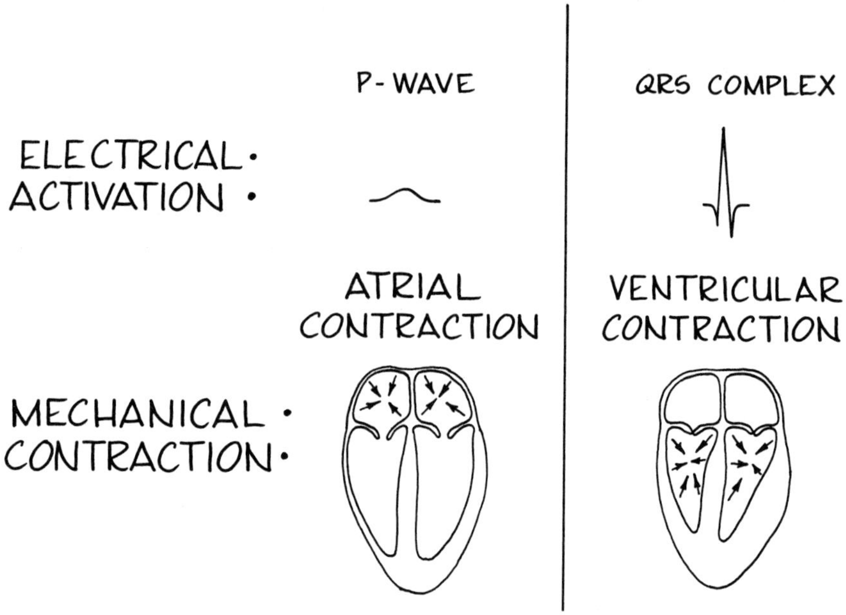

FIG 3–11.
Normal electromechanical coupling. Atrial depolarization (P wave) results in *atrial contraction;* ventricular depolarization (QRS complex) results in *ventricular contraction.*

ELECTROMECHANICAL COUPLING

Normally, electrical activation (depolarization) of muscle cells precedes mechanical contraction. This process is called *electromechanical coupling.* The electrical impulses (P wave and QRS complex) recorded in the ECG as *depolarization processes* slightly precede mechanical contraction of the atria and ventricles, respectively, in normal electromechanical coupling.

In certain clinical conditions, electrical impulses are recorded, but no mechanical contractions are produced. This situation is termed *electromechanical dissociation* (EMD). The causes of EMD inlude:

1. Myocardial infarction
2. Cardiac arrest
3. End-stage heart disease

In these situations, muscle cells are electrically activated, but are unable to undergo mechanical contraction.

Importantly, there are other clinical conditions that may be mistaken for electromechanical dissociation and require specific types of lifesaving therapies. These conditions include the following:

1. Severe blood loss
2. Marked volume depletion
3. Cardiac tamponade (fluid surrounding the heart)
4. Cardiac rupture

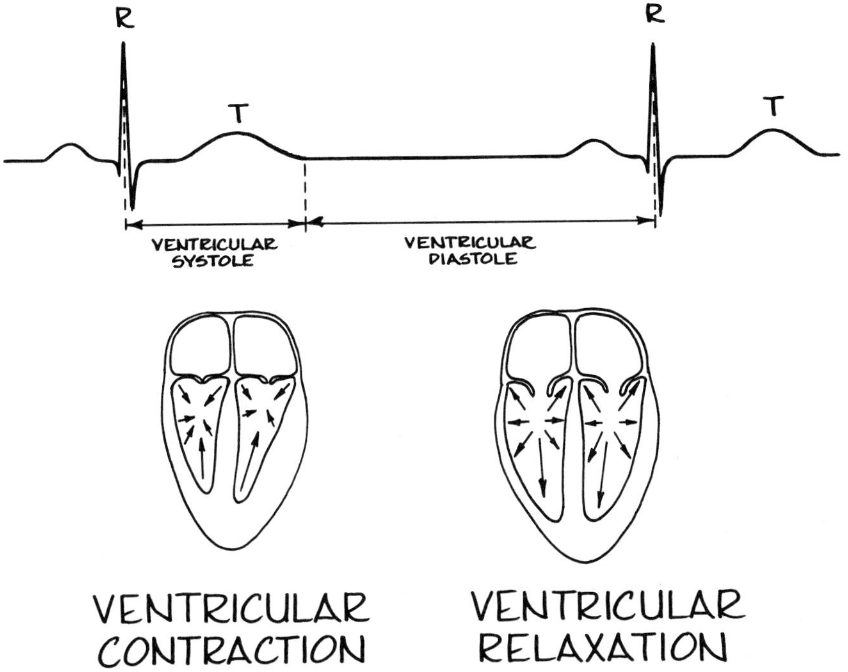

FIG 3–12.
Ventricular systole represents contraction of the ventricles, and in the ECG it occurs during the interval between the peak of the *R* wave and the end of the *T* wave. *Ventricular diastole* represents relaxation of the ventricles, and in the ECG it occurs during the remaining interval between the end of the *T* wave and the peak of the next *R* wave.

SYSTOLE AND DIASTOLE

The period during which mechanical contraction occurs is called *systole*. Atrial systole represents atrial contraction; ventricular systole represents ventricular contraction. The remaining periods of time during which the atria or ventricles are relaxing and filling with blood are called atrial *diastole* or ventricular *diastole*, respectively.

The figure shows the normal heartbeat recorded in the ECG. It also shows the periods of systole and diastole for the ventricles only. *Ventricular systole* (contraction) begins just after the onset of the QRS complex, near the peak of the R wave. *Ventricular diastole* (relaxation) begins after ventricular systole has been completed, usually at the end of the T wave, and continues to the peak of the next R wave.

Note that depolarization and repolarization are electrical processes. Systole and diastole are mechanical processes.

PEARLS

1. Determination of normal Q-T interval (Q-T corrected for heart rate) can also be done with a handy calculator:

$$\frac{\text{Q-T interval (in seconds)}}{\sqrt{\text{R-R interval (in seconds)}}}$$

Normal value for this ratio is less than 0.42.

2. Another rapid and accurate method to determine heart rate per minute is to count the number of *small squares* between two successive R waves and divide this number into 1,500.

3. Normal ECG findings and variations include the following:
   a. Negative P wave, QRS complex, and T wave in lead aVR
   b. Q wave and inverted T wave in lead III
   c. Biphasic P wave and inverted T wave in lead V_1
   d. Insignificant Q waves in leads I, aVL, V_5, V_6

4 / Axis

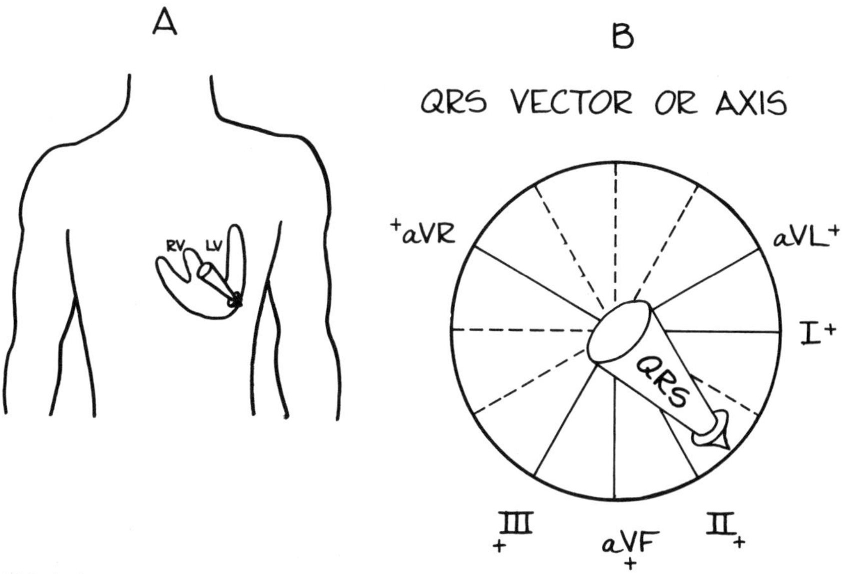

FIG 4–1.
A, the major direction of depolarization in the ventricles (mean QRS axis) represented by an *arrow* (vector). *LV,* left ventricle; *RV,* right ventricle. **B,** normal mean QRS vector or axis projected on the hexaxial reference system.

Axis is simply the major direction that the heart's electrical forces travel in relation to the frontal plane of the body. The major directions of the *depolarization* forces in the atria (mean P axis) or ventricles (mean QRS axis), as well as the major directions of the *repolarization* forces in the ventricles (mean ST axis, mean T axis), can be determined by examining the ECG.

Axis is an important ECG concept to understand, because many ECG diagnoses involve abnormalities in the axis.

The *mean QRS axis* is the major direction of the depolarization forces in the ventricles expressed as degrees on the hexaxial reference system (see Fig 2–6). Importantly, this main direction of ventricular depolarization can be altered by many causes, including hypertrophy of the ventricles, conduction blocks in the ventricles, myocardial infarction, COPD, preexcitation syndromes, and many other causes. Thus, determination of the mean QRS axis is important and should be routinely calculated in every ECG.

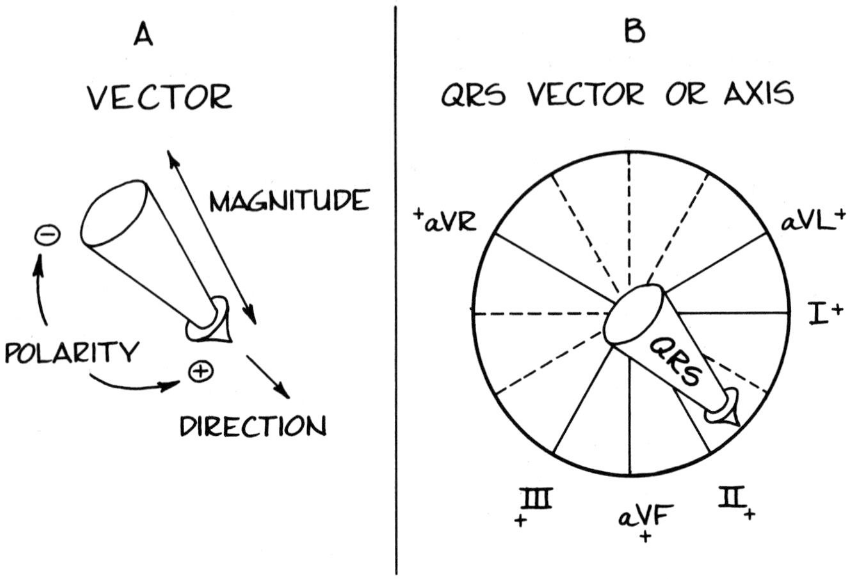

FIG 4–2.
A, *vector* drawn as an *arrow* representing *magnitude, direction,* and *polarity.* **B,** normal mean *QRS vector or axis* projected on the hexaxial reference system.

VECTOR AND AXIS

The concepts of vector and axis involve projecting the major direction of the heart's electrical forces recorded in the ECG onto the previously described *hexaxial reference system* (see Fig 2–6). A vector has *magnitude* (amount of electrical force), direction (which way the force travels), and *polarity* (positive and negative ends). A vector may be illustrated by an arrow; the length of the arrow represents magnitude of the electrical forces; the position of arrow represents direction; and the tip of the arrow represents the positive end, while the tail of arrow represents the negative end (Fig 4–2,*A*).

The P waves and QRS complexes are *depolarization forces;* the ST segments and T waves are *repolarization forces.* In the 12-lead ECG, the P, QRS, ST, and T wave deflections are electrical forces that can be represented by vectors. These vectors may be projected onto the hexaxial reference system to determine P, QRS, ST, or T axes.

The terms "vector" and "axis" are synonymous and may be used interchangeably. However, the term axis is preferable, and it refers to a vector that is placed on the hexaxial reference system (Fig 4–2,*B*).

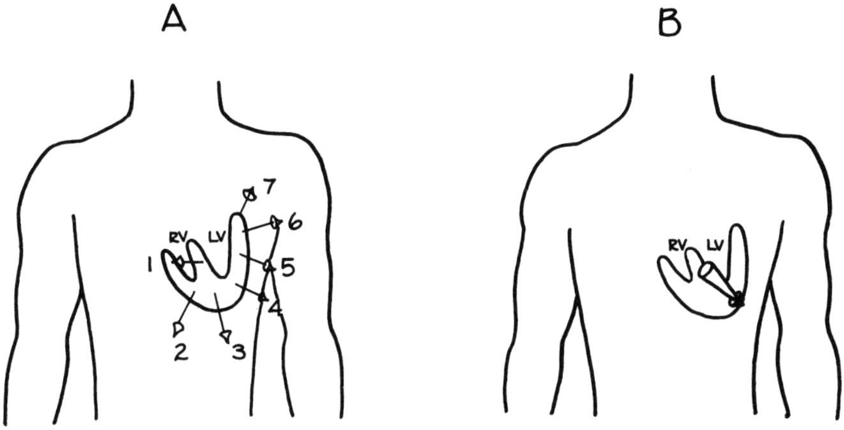

FIG 4–3.
A, instantaneous vectors of ventricular depolarization in sequence (*1* through *7*) during ventricular activation. **B,** normal mean *QRS* vector or axis representing average of all the instantaneous QRS vectors (frontal view). *RV,* right ventricle; *LV,* left venticle.

QRS AXIS

Determination of *QRS axis* (axis of ventricular depolarization), as opposed to P, ST, or T axes, will be discussed in the remainder of the chapter. As the ventricles are depolarized, multiple small instantaneous vectors are present (Fig 4–3,*A*). The *mean QRS vector* or *mean QRS axis* is the average of these small instantaneous vectors. *The mean QRS vector represents the main direction of depolarization in the ventricles.*

Normally, the left ventricle is much larger than the right; thus, the left ventricle is responsible for most of the heart's electrical forces. The major direction of ventricular depolarization (mean QRS axis) normally points toward the left side of the patient's body, as well as downward and posteriorly. When viewed from the front of the body (frontal plane), the mean QRS axis points to the left and downward (Fig 4–3,*B*).

RELATION OF ECG LEADS TO AXIS LEADS

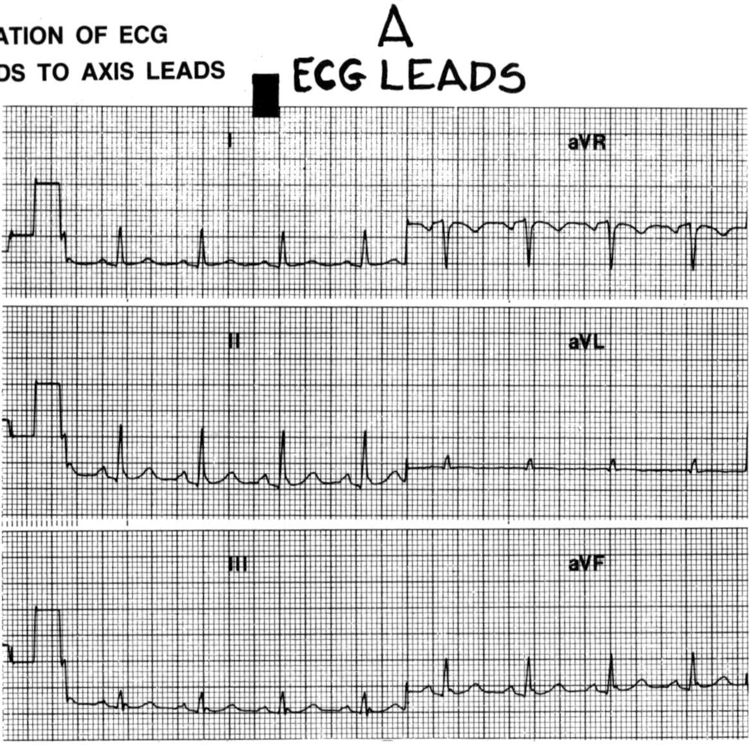

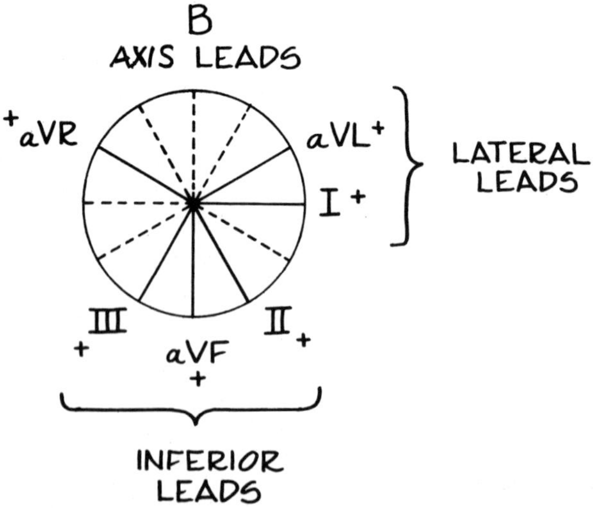

FIG 4–4.
A, the six-*limb ECG leads: I, II, III, aVR, aVL, aVF.* **B,** the six-*limb axis leads* in the hexaxial reference system. Note that the *solid lines* indicate the positive (+) ends of the axis leads; the *dotted lines* indicate the negative (−) ends of the axis leads. The inferior leads are II, III, aVF; the lateral leads are I, aVL.

RELATION OF ECG LEADS TO AXIS LEADS

The hexaxial reference system is comprised of the three standard limb leads (I, II, III) and the three unipolar limb leads (aVR, aVL, aVF). Each *ECG lead* (Fig 4–4,*A*), when transposed onto the hexaxial system, is called an *axis lead* (formerly "lead axis") (Fig 4–4,*B*). As an example, *ECG lead* I, when projected onto the hexaxial reference system, is called *axis lead* I. Each *axis lead* has a positive (+) and a negative (−) end corresponding to the positive and negative ends of its respective *ECG lead* (see Fig 2–6).

In the hexaxial reference system, specific leads represent certain areas of the heart. For example, the leads that record the undersurface or *inferior* area of the heart are leads II, III, aVF. These leads are called the *inferior leads*. The leads that record the left side or *lateral* area of the heart are I and aVL. These leads are called the *lateral leads*. Electrical changes in these groups of leads localize changes in those respective areas of the heart (see location of myocardial infarction, Fig 7–5).

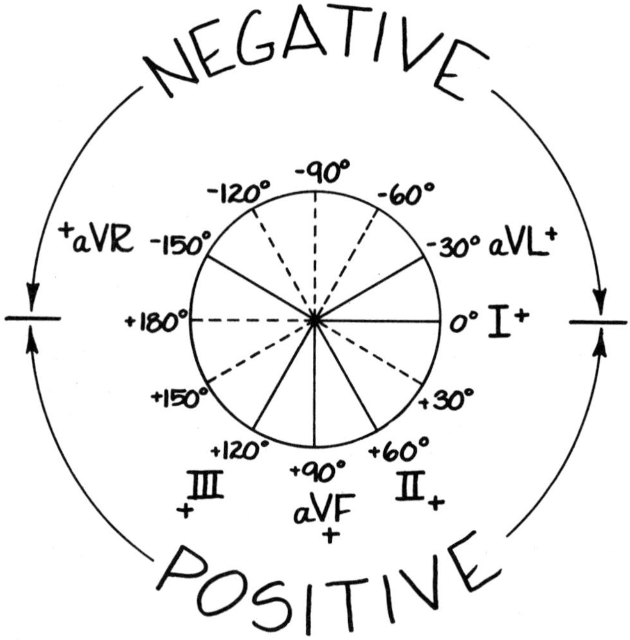

FIG 4–5.
The hexaxial reference system enclosed in a 360° circle. The location of each end of an axis lead corresponds to a specific degree on the circle. The upper half of the circle is marked in *negative* degrees, the lower half in *positive* degrees.

AXIS LEADS AND CORRESPONDING DEGREES ON THE HEXAXIAL REFERENCE SYSTEM

The hexaxial reference system is enclosed in a circle (360°) divided by the six *axis leads*. The upper 180° (upper half of the circle) is negative; the lower 180° (lower half) is positive. Each end of an axis lead corresponds to a particular degree on the hexaxial reference system.

The location of the positive ends of the axis leads on the hexaxial reference system are important to remember. The *positive* ends of the standard limb leads are projected as *axis leads* on the reference system as follows: I is 0°, II is +60°, III is +120°. They are separated by 60° intervals in a clockwise direction.

The *positive* ends of the unipolar limb leads are projected as *axis leads* on the reference system as follows: aVF is +90°, aVL is −30°, aVR is −150°. Imagine looking at a person whose arms are held slightly above the shoulders. Then, aVR is right arm (−150°), aVL is left arm (−30°), and aVF is left foot (+90°). They are separated by 120° intervals.

The final *mean QRS axis* viewed from the frontal plane of the body is expressed as a specific degree on this hexaxial reference system.

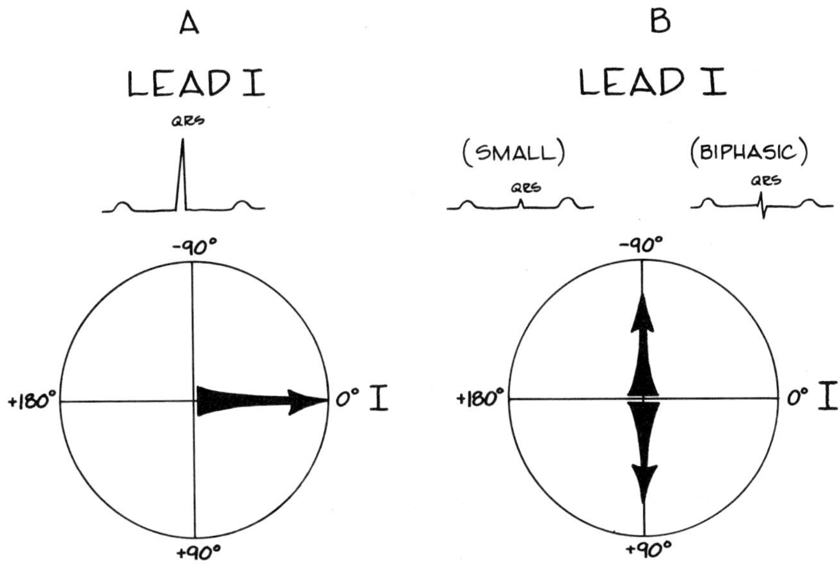

FIG 4–6.
A, the large, positive QRS deflection in *ECG lead I* projects on the hexaxial reference system as a vector that points toward the positive end of *axis lead I.* **B,** a *small* or *biphasic* QRS deflection in *ECG lead I* projects as a vector that points perpendicular to *axis lead I.* Note that the vector in this case can be directed perpendicular to either side of *axis lead I.*

DETERMINATION OF QRS VECTOR

The QRS vector is determined from the ECG by projecting the magnitude, direction, and polarity of the QRS deflection in the *ECG lead* onto its *axis lead* in the hexaxial reference system. If the majority of the QRS deflection in the *ECG lead* is above the baseline (positive), the vector will point toward the positive (+) end of that *axis lead.* However, if the majority of the QRS deflection in the *ECG lead* is below the baseline (negative), the vector will point toward the negative (−) end of that *axis lead* in the reference system. If there is little or no QRS deflection *or* if there is the same amount of positive as negative QRS deflection (biphasic) in the *ECG lead,* the vector will be perpendicular to that *axis lead* in the reference system.

It is important to remember that the *largest* deflection in an *ECG lead* projects a vector that is *parallel* to its corresponding *axis lead.* Conversely, the *smallest* or *biphasic* QRS deflection in an *ECG lead* projects a vector that is *perpendicular* to its correponding *axis lead.*

For example, if the QRS deflection in *ECG lead* I is predominantly upright (positive), the vector points to the positive side of *axis lead* I (Fig 4–6,A). If the QRS deflection in ECG lead I is small or biphasic, the vector points perpendicular to *axis lead* I in the reference system (Fig 4–6,*B*).

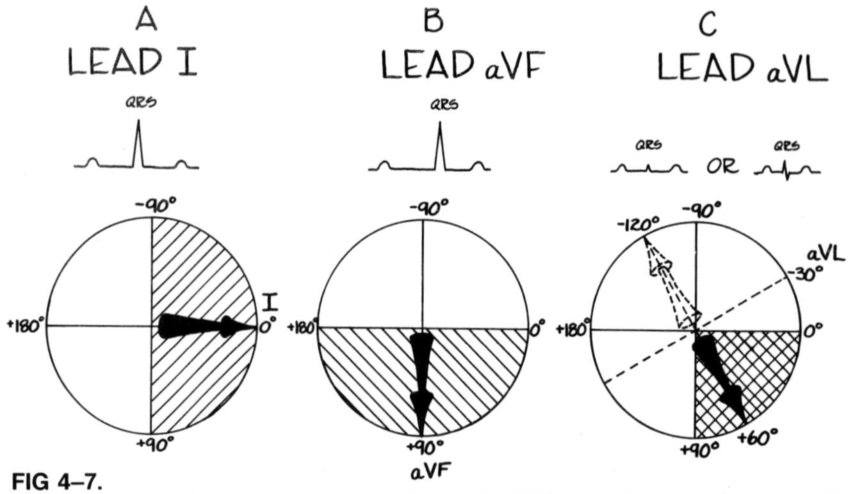

FIG 4–7.
A, projection of the positive QRS deflection in *ECG lead I* onto *axis lead I.* **B,** projection of the positive QRS deflection in *ECG lead aVF* onto *axis lead aVF.* **C,** projection of the small or biphasic QRS deflection in *ECG lead aVL* perpendicular to both sides of *axis lead aVL.* The correct mean QRS axis is +60°, which lies between 0° and +90° as previously determined by the vectors in *I* and *aVF.*

DETERMINATION OF MEAN QRS AXIS

The *mean QRS axis* represents the main direction of depolarization in the ventricles. A simple method of determining mean QRS axis is by projecting the predominate QRS deflections in two ECG *limb leads* as vectors onto their respective *axis leads* in the hexaxial reference system and then averaging the two vectors.

As an example, if the QRS deflection in *ECG lead* I is primarily positive, the vector points toward the positive side of *axis lead* I, toward 0° in the reference system (Fig 4–7,*A*). *In the same ECG,* if the QRS deflection in *ECG lead* aVF is primarily positive, the vector points toward the positive side of *axis lead* aVF, toward +90° in the reference system (Fig 4–7,*B*). When these two vectors are averaged, the *mean* QRS axis points somewhere in between these two vectors; i.e., the mean QRS axis will lie between 0° and +90°.

To localize more accurately the mean QRS axis, find the *ECG lead* with the smallest or biphasic QRS deflection. When that *ECG lead* is found, the final mean QRS axis is perpendicular to that *axis lead* in the reference system. In the example (Fig 4–7,*C*), the QRS deflection in *ECG lead* aVL is small or biphasic. The mean QRS axis thus lies perpendicular to *axis lead* aVL. The axis points toward +60° or −120°; both directions are perpendicular to *axis lead* aVL. However, the mean QRS axis of +60° is the correct one, because it lies between 0° and +90° as previously determined.

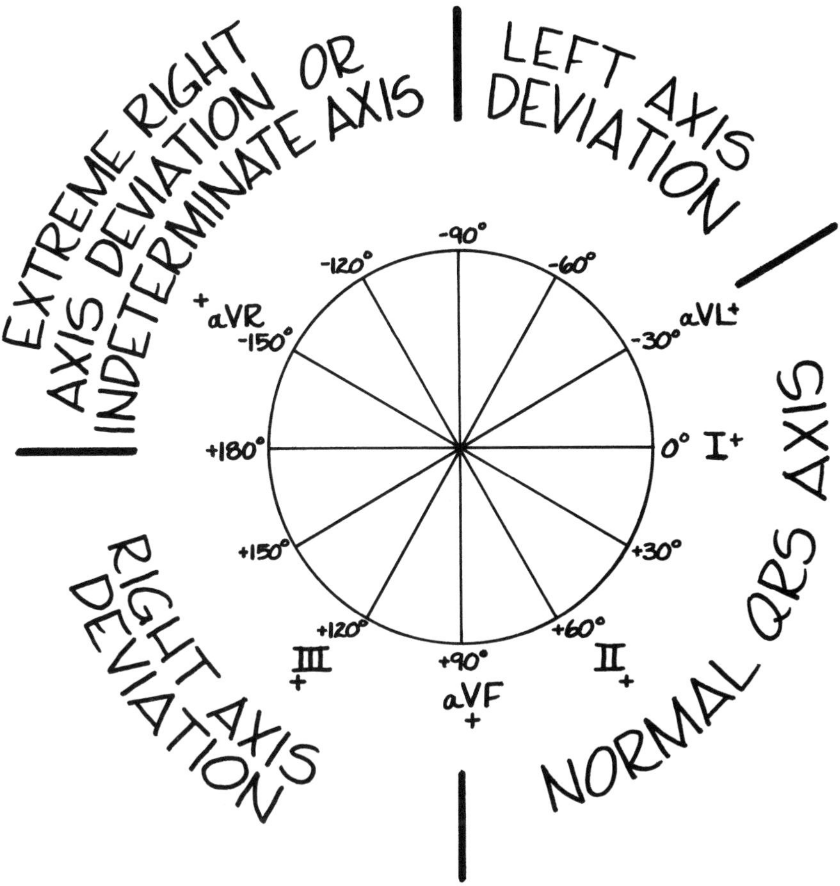

FIG 4–8.
QRS axis deviation. Normal mean QRS axis lies between +*90*° and −*30*°. *Right axis deviation* lies between +90° and +180°. *Left axis deviation* lies between −*30*° and −*90*°. *Indeterminate* or *extreme right axis deviation* lies between −90° and +*180*°.

QRS AXIS DEVIATION

The mean QRS axis is projected onto the hexaxial reference system and is expressed in degrees. As stated previously, the normal ventricular depolarization vector projects to the left and downward in the frontal plane (see Fig 4–3,*B*). The range of *normal mean QRS axis* lies between +90° and −30° in the hexaxial reference system (see above figure).

Axis deviation is present when the mean QRS axis lies outside of the normal range. *Left axis deviation* (LAD) is present when the mean QRS axis lies between −30° and −90°. *Right axis deviation* (RAD) is present when the mean QRS axis lies between +90° and +180°. The remaining left upper quadrant between +180° and −90° is referred to as extreme RAD or indeterminate axis.

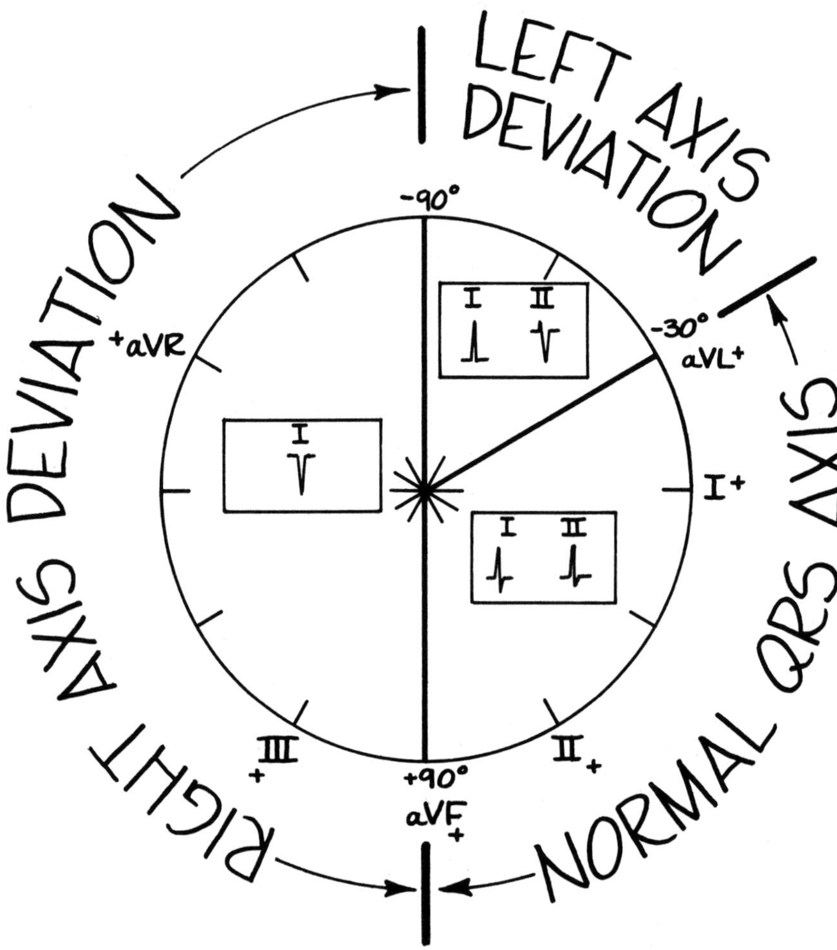

FIG 4–9.
Rapid estimation of mean QRS axis using only ECG leads *I* and *II*. *Normal QRS axis* is present when the QRS complexes in leads *I* and *II* are positive. *Left axis deviation* is present when the QRS in lead *I* is positive and the QRS in lead *II* is negative. *Right axis deviation* occurs when the QRS in lead *I* is negative regardless of lead *II*.

RAPID ESTIMATION OF MEAN QRS AXIS

By scanning the main QRS deflections in ECG leads I and II, the mean QRS axis may be rapidly estimated (see Fig 4–9):

	Main QRS Deflection	
	Lead I	Lead II
Normal QRS axis	Positive	Positive
Left axis deviation	Positive	Negative
Right axis deviation	Negative	(Unnecessary)

For a more accurate determination of QRS axis, when the quadrant in the hexaxial reference system is found, find the ECG lead with the smallest or biphasic QRS deflection. The mean QRS axis is *perpendicular* to that axis lead in that quadrant in the reference system.

PEARLS

1. Causes of LAD include the following:
   a. Normal variant
   b. Left anterior fascicular block (LAFB)
   c. Older age
   d. Left ventricular hypertrophy (LVH)
   e. Chronic obstructive lung disease (COPD)
   f. Inferior myocardial infarction
   g. Preexcitation syndromes (Wolff-Parkinson-White syndrome)
2. Causes of RAD include the following:
   a. Normal variant
   b. Left posterior fascicular block (LPFB)
   c. Younger age (infants and children)
   d. Right ventricular hypertrophy (RVH)
   e. COPD
   f. Lateral myocardial infarction
   g. Preexcitation syndromes (Wolff-Parkinson-White syndrome)
3. A simple way to check for reversed limb electrodes is to observe the QRS voltage. If the limb electrodes are placed correctly, the QRS voltage in lead I plus the QRS voltage in lead III equals the QRS voltage in lead II.

5 / Arrhythmias

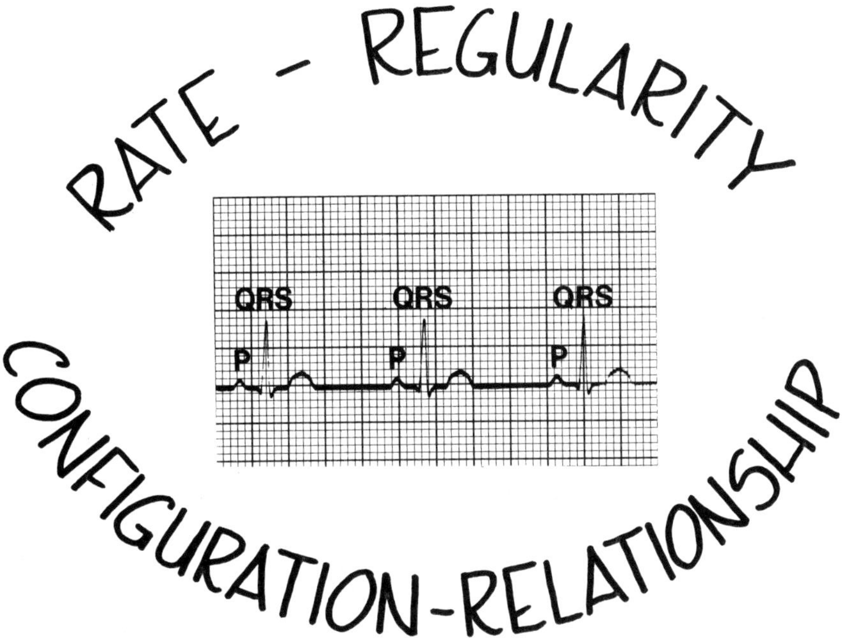

FIG 5–1.
Rhythms are determined by evaluating the *rate, regularity, configuration,* and *relationship* of *P* waves and *QRS* complexes.

The ECG is especially useful in the diagnosis of arrhythmias. An arrhythmia is any rhythm other than a normal sinus rhythm. Many arrhythmias are harmless, depending upon the clinical situation. However, some arrhythmias may be life-threatening if the heart is unable to maintain adequate circulation.

Rhythms are determined by examining four basic aspects in the ECG:

1. *Rate* of P waves (P-P intervals) and QRS complexes (R-R intervals)
2. *Regularity* of P waves and QRS complexes
3. *Configuration* of P waves and QRS complexes
4. *Relation* of P waves to QRS complexes

When analyzing rhythms, first search for the P waves. They are best seen in the inferior leads (II, III, aVF) or chest leads V_1, V_2. If P waves are not readily identifiable in a 12-lead ECG, *Lewis* leads, esophageal leads, or intra-atrial leads may be used to identify P waves (see p. 73). The QRS complexes are usually easily visualized. Once the P waves and QRS complexes are identified, the rate, regularity, configuration, and relation of both are correlated to determine the rhythm.

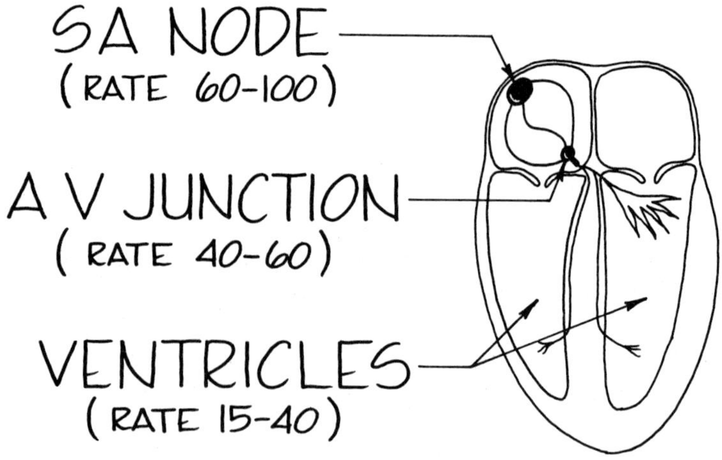

FIG 5–2.
Pacemaker sites in the heart and their normal intrinsic rates of discharge. *SA,* sinoatrial; *AV,* atrioventricular.

PACEMAKER SITES

The SA node, located high in the right atrium, is the pacemaker site where impulses are normally initiated. Impulses originating outside of the SA node are termed "ectopic." If the SA node fails, either a lower escape pacemaker site takes over, or the heart stops beating. Potential ectopic pacemaker sites are located throughout the heart in the atria, AV junction, and the ventricles.

Normally, pacemaker cells in the SA node have the fastest resting rate of discharge at a rate of 60–100 beats/min in adults. Lower ectopic pacemaker sites have a slower intrinsic rate. When a higher pacemaker site fails to discharge, a lower site normally takes over. This is termed *escape* rhythm.

The junctional area surrounding the AV node normally has an intrinsic rate of 40–60 beats/min. If the ectopic impulses originate in this area as an escape rhythm, it is termed a *junctional escape rhythm.* Ventricular pacemaker cells possess an intrinsic rate of 15–40 beats/min. If the ectopic impulses originate in the ventricles as an escape rhythm, it is called a *ventricular escape rhythm.*

Rarely, a lower ectopic pacemaker site may increase its rate and *usurp* the normal sinus rhythm. For example, an enhanced junctional pacemaker may fire at a rate greater than 60 beats/min and override the SA node (accelerated junctional rhythm, see Fig 5–11). This may occur in digoxin toxicity ("Dig. toxicity") and acute myocardial infarction.

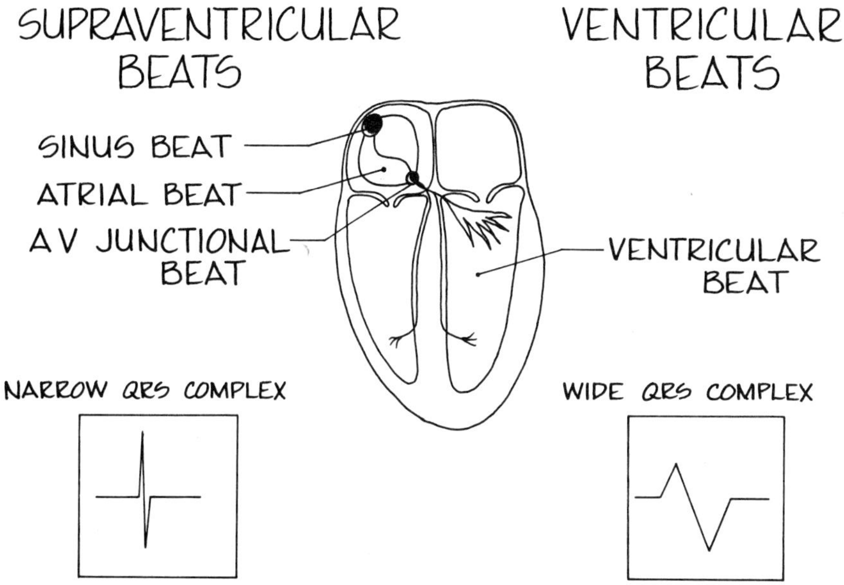

FIG 5–3.
Supraventricular beats originate above the ventricles and are usually characterized by narrow QRS complexes (normal ventricular conduction). Ventricular beats originate in the ventricles and are characterized by wide QRS complexes (abnormal ventricular conduction).

SUPRAVENTRICULAR AND VENTRICULAR ARRHYTHMIAS

Arrhythmias may be divided into two broad categories: supraventricular and ventricular. In *supraventricular* arrhythmias, the pacemaker impulses originate above the ventricles ("supra," prefix meaning above). It includes pacemaker sites in the SA node, the atria, the AV junction, and the bundle of His. Supraventricular impulses usually depolarize the ventricles through normal conduction pathways described previously, which produce *narrow* QRS complexes. The hallmark of a supraventricular beat is a narrow, normal-appearing QRS complex (for exceptions see p. 48).

In *ventricular* arrhythmias, the pacemaker impulses originate in the ventricles. Depolarization of the ventricles occurs in a slow, random fashion (muscle cell to muscle cell) as opposed to an organized manner through the normal ventricular conduction pathways. This abnormal depolarization produces a *wide* QRS complex with a QRS duration greater than 0.12 second. The hallmark of a ventricular beat is a wide bizarre QRS complex.

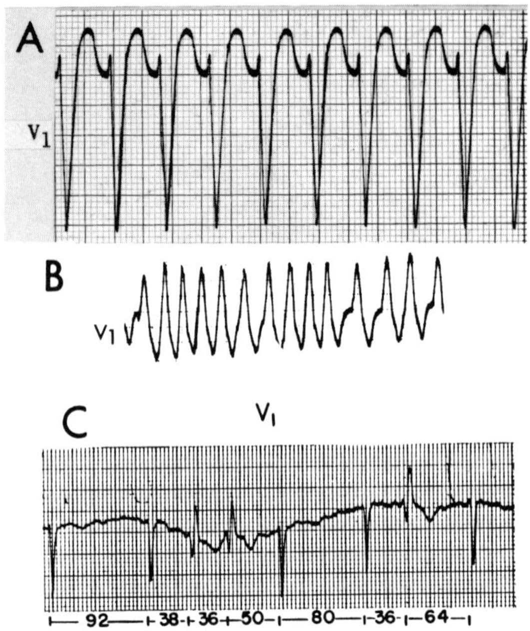

FIG 5–4.
A, supraventricular tachycardia with wide QRS complexes at a rate of 172 beats/min in a patient with preexisting LBBB. **B,** wide QRS complex tachycardia with a rapid, irregular rate (between 180 and 230 beats/min.) This is atrial fibrillation in a patient with Wolff-Parkinson-White syndrome. The rapid, irregular supraventricular impulses conduct to the ventricles through the accessory pathway, producing the wide QRS complexes. This is often mistaken for ventricular tachycardia. **C,** atrial fibrillation, supraventricular rhythm, with aberration. The aberrant ventricular beats (Ashman beats) have a wider QRS duration and a shorter cycle length than the normally conducted ventricular beats.

SUPRAVENTRICULAR RHYTHM WITH WIDE QRS COMPLEXES

Importantly, *supraventricular* impulses may at times conduct through the ventricles in an altered or abnormal fashion resulting in wide, bizarre QRS complexes that are difficult to distinguish from ventricular-initiated ectopic impulses. There are three main causes for wide QRS complexes that originate from supraventricular sites, but look like ventricular ectopic beats: (1) *bundle branch block* (see p. 85), (2) *preexcitation syndromes* (see pp. 136 and 137), (3) *aberrant ventricular conduction* (see p. 139). Criteria for differentiating the origin of wide, bizarre QRS complex tachycardias (supraventricular vs. ventricular) are discussed on p. 141.

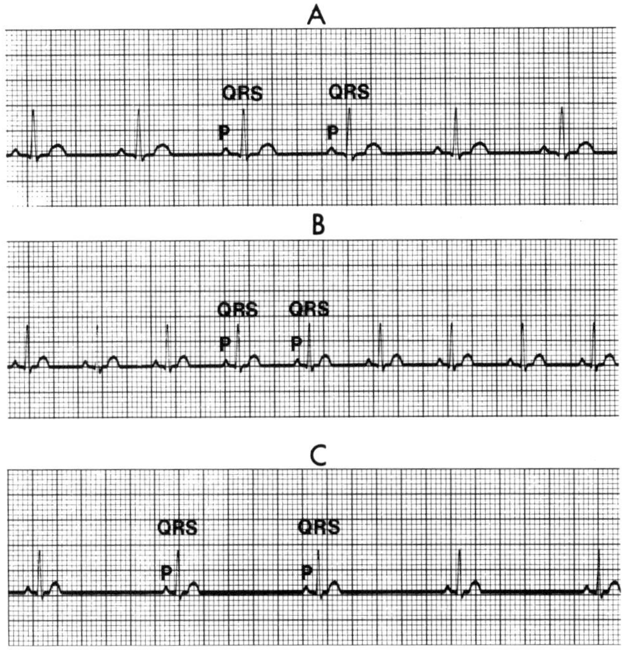

FIG 5–5.
A, normal sinus rhythm at a rate of 72 beats/min. **B,** sinus tachycardia at a rate of 104 beats/min. **C,** sinus bradycardia at a rate of 54 beats/min.

NORMAL SINUS RHYTHM

Sinus Tachycardia, Sinus Bradycardia

In *normal sinus rhythm,* the pacemaker impulse is initiated in the SA node and passes through the atrial internodal pathways to the AV node. Atrial depolarization produces a normal P wave. From the AV node, conduction proceeds through the ventricular conduction system, resulting in ventricular depolarization and the QRS complex. In normal sinus rhythm (Fig 5–5,*A*), the ECG displays a normal P wave followed by a QRS complex. Usually, the P-P and R-R intervals are constant and equal at a rate of 60–100 beats/min. The normal P-R interval is 0.12–0.20 second.

Arbitrarily, tachycardia is any rate greater than 100 beats/min; bradycardia is any rate less than 60 beats/min. *Sinus tachycardia* (Fig 5–5,*B*) denotes a sinus rhythm that is initiated in the SA node at a rate greater than 100 beats/min. *Sinus bradycardia* (Fig 5–5,*C*) denotes a sinus rhythm that is initiated in the SA node at a rate less than 60 beats/min.

SINUS ARRHYTHMIA

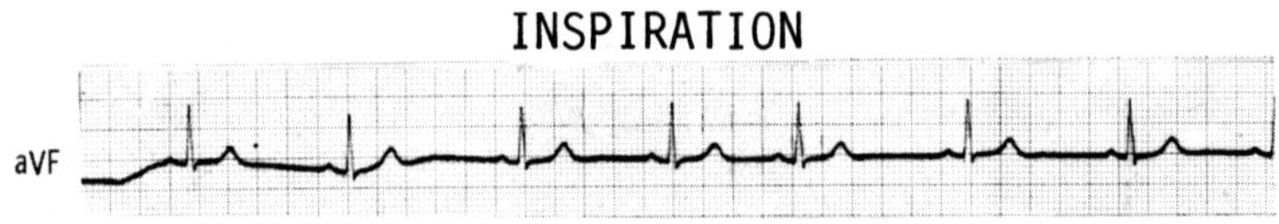

FIG 5–6.
Sinus arrhythmia. Rate increases with inspiration and decreases with expiration. Note the shorter P–P intervals (and P-R intervals) during inspiration.

SINUS ARRHYTHMIA

Sinus arrhythmia is a sinus rhythm with a rate that varies slightly with respirations. During inspiration, heart rate increases; during expiration, heart rate decreases. The variations in heart rate are denoted by varying P-P intervals. The P wave, P-R interval, and QRS complex remain unchanged. This rhythm is benign and is commonly found in children and young adults.

Occasionally in adult patients with heart disease or after inferior myocardial infarction, a *nonrespiratory sinus arrhythmia* may occur. Moreover, enhanced vagal tone and drugs such as digoxin may cause this type of sinus arrhythmia.

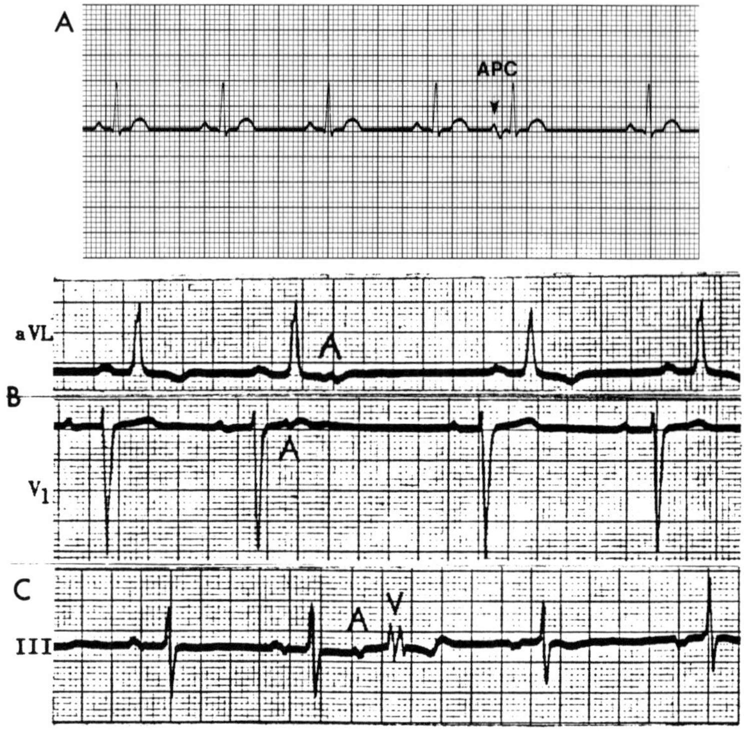

FIG 5–7.
Atrial premature contraction *(APC)*. An abnormal P wave *(APC)* precedes the early QRS complex. A normal QRS follows the APC. **B,** blocked or nonconducted atrial premature contractions *(A)* deforming the preceding T wave. No QRS follows these very early APCs due to *complete refractoriness* of the junctional and ventricular pathways, resulting in the *nonconducted, blocked* APCs. This pause is the most common cause of a lengthened cycle for which a reason is not obvious at first glance. **C,** atrial premature contraction *(A')* followed by a long PR and an aberrant QRS–due to *partial refractoriness* in the junctional and ventricular pathways.

ATRIAL PREMATURE CONTRACTION

Atrial premature contraction (APC) is an ectopic, supraventricular impulse that originates *in the atria* outside of the SA node. Atrial depolarization from an APC does not proceed through the normal atrial conduction pathways. Thus, the P wave assumes a bizarre or inverted configuration. Because the atrial impulse occurs early, the premature P wave may coincide with or distort the T wave of the previous beat. Importantly, an abnormal or notched T wave preceding an early QRS complex may often be a helpful clue in diagnosing an APC (Fig 5–7,*B*).

The QRS complex following an APC usually remains similar in configuration to the QRS complex of previous sinus beats, because conduction through the ventricles is unchanged. However, if the APC occurs very early, the ventricles may be *partially refractory* to depolarization because some parts of the ventricles may not have fully repolarized from the previous sinus beat. In this instance, the premature P wave will be followed by a slightly slurred or widened QRS complex, because the usual sequence of ventricular depolarization is altered (see Fig 5–7,*C*). This phenomenon is termed *ventricular aberrancy* (see Fig 9–19,A). If the premature P wave occurs too early, the ventricles may be *totally refractory* to depolarization. In this instance, the P wave will *not* be followed by a QRS complex. This is known as a *nonconducted or blocked APC*, which is the commonest cause of a pause during normal sinus rhythm (see Fig 5–7,*B*).

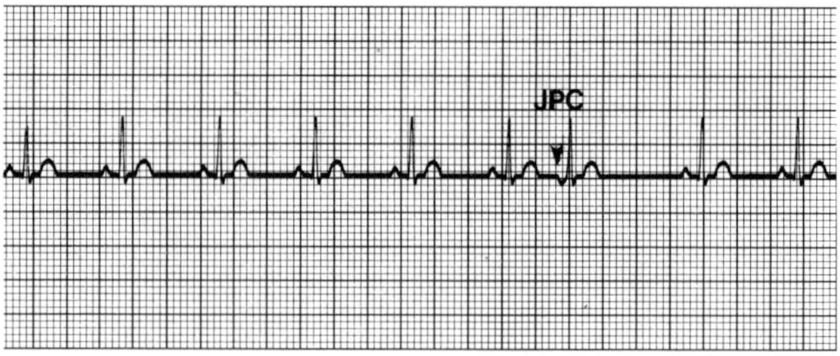

FIG 5–8.
Junctional premature contraction *(JPC).* An inverted P wave immediately precedes the early QRS complex.

JUNCTIONAL PREMATURE CONTRACTION

There are no pacemaking cells located in the center of the AV node itself. However, pacemaking cells do exist at the junctions located just above and below the AV node. Thus, impulses arising from this area are known as *AV junctional* or simply *junctional* beats.

Junctional premature contraction (JPC) is an ectopic, supraventricular impulse that originates in the AV junction. A P wave may or may not be identified, depending on whether there is *retrograde* (backward) conduction to the atria. If retrograde atrial conduction occurs, the P wave will assume an abnormal configuration, usually inverted, in leads II, III, aVF. This P wave may occur just before or just after the QRS complex (depending on the rate of retrograde atrial conduction), or the P wave may be buried in the QRS complex and not seen at all. The contour of the QRS complex of a JPC usually remains similar to that of previous sinus beats, because conduction through the ventricles is unchanged.

A JPC is usually recognized by a premature QRS complex, which *may or may not* have an inverted P wave just preceding or just following it. The occurrence of JPCs is much less frequent than that of APCs.

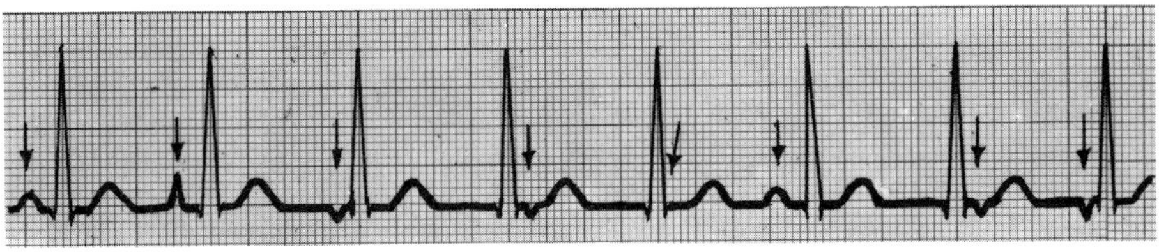

FIG 5–9.
Wandering atrial pacemaker between the SA node and the AV junction. More than two different atrial foci with varying P wave configurations and P-R intervals discharge at a rate of 75 beats/min.

WANDERING ATRIAL PACEMAKER

Wandering atrial pacemaker is a supraventricular rhythm where the pacemaker impulses originate from two or more different foci in the SA node, atria, or AV junction at a rate between 60 and 100 beats/min. Depolarization of the atria proceeds from these different foci to produce P waves of varying configurations and varying P-R intervals. The varying P wave contours represent the different pathways taken by the impulses to depolarize the atria.

In wandering atrial pacemaker, the following occur:

1. P wave configurations and P-R intervals vary because of the different atrial pacemaker sites and disordered pathways of atrial depolarization
2. The average rate is between 60 and 100 beats/min.
3. QRS complexes are usually identical because of unchanged conduction in the ventricles.

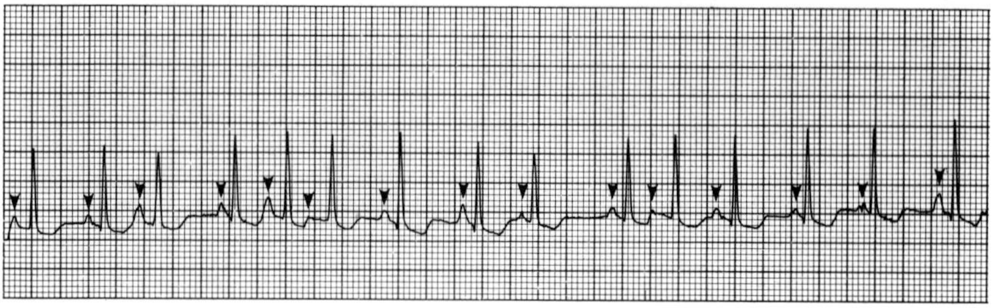

FIG 5–10.
Multifocal atrial tachycardia. Greater than three different atrial foci *(arrows)* discharge irregularly at a rate between 90 and 180 beats/min.

MULTIFOCAL ATRIAL TACHYCARDIA

Multifocal atrial tachycardia (MAT) is a supraventricular tachycardia that originates from three or more different ectopic atrial foci at a rate between 100 and 250 beats/min. The mechanism is believed to be enhanced automaticity of ectopic atrial pacemakers.

The ECG criteria for MAT are as follows:

1. Three or more different ectopic atrial foci producing three or more different P wave configurations and varying P-R intervals.
2. Varying P-P intervals (P waves occur irregularly).
3. Tachycardia, rate between 100 and 250 beats/min.

Conduction usually proceeds unchanged through the ventricles to produce identical QRS complexes. If an early P wave occurs, the ventricles may be *partially refractory* and produce slightly slurred or widened QRS complexes because of *aberrant ventricular conduction* (see Fig 9–19,*A*).

Usually MAT is found in patients with COPD and acute respiratory distress with resulting hypoxemia (decreased arterial Po_2). Treatment is correction of hypoxemia or other underlying causes.

Note that if P waves are not readily identifiable, MAT may resemble atrial fibrillation (see Fig 5–14).

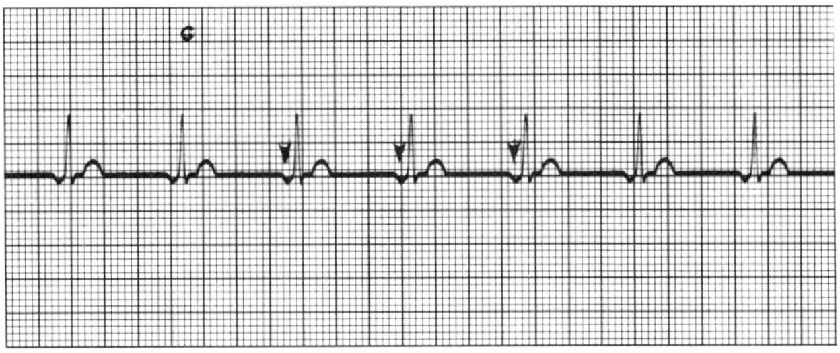

FIG 5–11.
Accelerated junctional rhythm. Note the inverted *P* waves *(arrows)* immediately preceding the narrow QRS complexes at a rate of 95 beats/min. The inverted *P* waves represent retrograde atrial conduction from the enhanced junctional pacemaker site.

ACCELERATED JUNCTIONAL RHYTHM

Accelerated junctional rhythm is a supraventricular rhythm that originates from an enhanced focus in the AV junction at a rate faster than the normal intrinsic junctional rate of 40–60 beats/min. The QRS complexes are usually narrow and unchanged in configuration and occur at a rate of 60–150 beats/min. If there is retrograde conduction from the junctional pacemaker to the atria, inverted P waves may be seen in leads II, III, aVF. The P waves may occur just before or after the QRS complexes (see above) or may be hidden in the QRS complexes and not seen at all.

The mechanism of impulse formation in accelerated junctional rhythm is an enhanced automatic focus in the AV junction that usurps SA node activity and fires at a rate between 60 and 150 beats/min. This rhythm is also known as *nonparoxysmal junctional tachycardia,* which should be distinguished from *paroxysmal junctional tachycardia,* which involves a reentry circuit as its mechanism of impulse formation (see pp. 58 and 135).

Accelerated junctional rhythm (nonparoxysmal junctional tachycardia) may begin abruptly and persist for longer periods of time than paroxysmal junctional tachycardia. It usually occurs in patients with heart disease and is one type of AV dissociation (see Fig 5–27,*B*). The two most common causes of accelerated junctional rhythm are "Dig. toxicity" and acute inferior myocardial infarction.

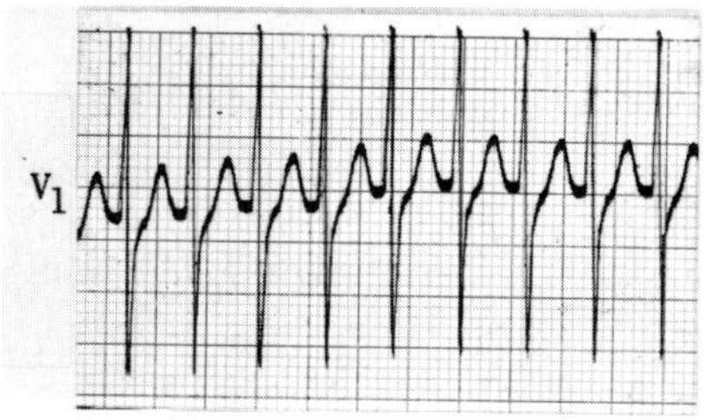

FIG 5–12.
Paroxysmal atrial tachycardia. The rate is 225 beats/min, and the retrograde P waves are not seen. The most common mechanism is a reentry circuit in the AV junction.

PAROXYSMAL ATRIAL TACHYCARDIA

Paroxysmal atrial tachycardia (PAT) refers to a supraventricular tachycardia derived from impulses that follow a *reentry circuit* in the atria or in the AV junctional area. A reentry circuit implies a closed loop or circular path through which an impulse continuously follows itself (see p. 135). The arrhythmia starts abruptly, ends abruptly, and conducts impulses to the ventricles at a rate between 150 and 250 beats/min.

The reentry circuit causing PAT may be located in the SA node (sinus node reentrant tachycardia), in the atria (intra-atrial reentrant tachycardia), or in the AV junction (AV junctional reentrant tachycardia). *The most frequent mechanism of PAT is a reentry circuit in the AV junction; AV junctional reentrant tachycardia is also known as paroxysmal junctional tachycardia.*

Usually PAT is initiated by an APC that has a longer-than-normal P-R interval. The reentry circuit conducts impulses to the ventricles at a rate between 150 and 250 beats/min, usually producing narrow QRS complexes. Retrograde P waves are frequently hidden in the QRS complexes.

Abrupt onset and termination characterize PAT. If it does not cease spontaneously, vagal maneuvers such as carotid sinus massage, valsalva, or diving reflex (immersing face in cold water) may be used to terminate the rhythm when the reentry circuit is in the AV junction. Drugs used to terminate this rhythm include calcium channel blockers, digoxin, β-blockers, and others.

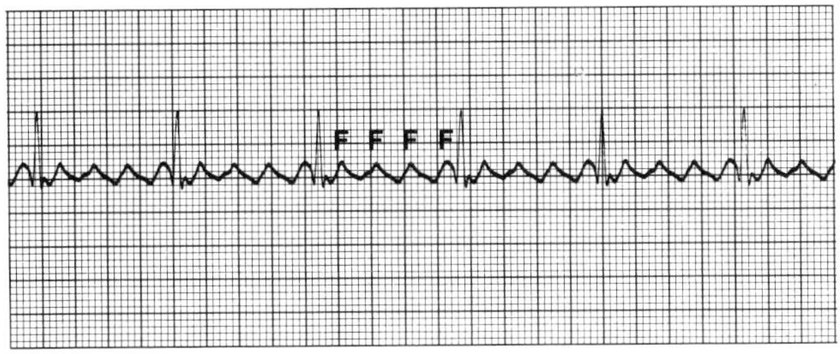

FIG 5–13.
Atrial flutter. Note the characteristic saw-tooth pattern of the flutter *(F)* waves at a rate of 300 beats/min. There is 4:1 A:V conduction resulting in a ventricular rate of about 75 beats/min.

ATRIAL FLUTTER

Atrial flutter is a supraventricular tachycardia that originates in the atria. The ECG displays *flutter* (F) waves that have the configuration of a saw-tooth or picket fence pattern with no baseline seen between the F waves. It is a rapid, regular rhythm with F waves occurring at a rate between 250 and 350 beats/min. The F waves are seen best in leads II, III, aVF, or V_1.

The ventricular rate (R-R interval) is determined by the rate of conduction of these atrial impulses through the AV node. The AV node does not normally conduct at a rate greater than 175 beats/min. When the atrial rate is 250–350 beats/min, the ventricular rate will be a *multiple* of the atrial rate. In other words, the ratio of atrial to ventricular conduction (A:V ratio) will be 2:1, 3:1, 4:1, etc., depending on how many supraventricular impulses the AV node conducts to the ventricles. Because conduction through the ventricles proceeds unchanged, QRS complexes will be unchanged in configuration. If conduction to the ventricles is too fast, the QRS complexes may become slightly slurred or widened from *aberrant conduction* (see p. 139).

In atrial flutter, the following occur:

1. Flutter waves are best seen in leads II, III, aVF, and V_1.
2. Atrial rate is usually 300 beats/min, but may vary between 250 and 350 beats/min.
3. Ventricular rate is a multiple of atrial rate, usually an even multiple: 2:1, 4:1, etc.

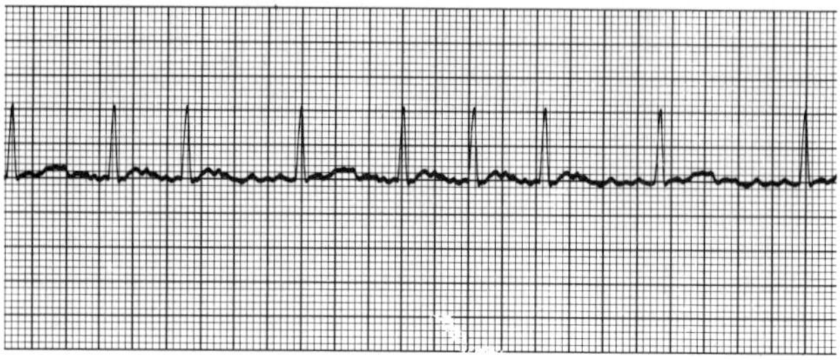

FIG 5–14.
Atrial fibrillation. Note the irregular oscillations of the baseline with no discreet P waves. The ventricular rate is irregularly irregular and varies between 70 and 140 beats/min.

ATRIAL FIBRILLATION

Atrial fibrillation is a supraventricular tachycardia characterized by (1) absent P waves and (2) irregularly irregular R-R intervals (variable ventricular rate). Impulses originate from multiple ectopic atrial sites at a rate of 350–600 impulses/min, producing irregular, coarse, or fine undulations of the ECG baseline, as opposed to the discrete P waves that are seen in normal sinus rhythm. These undulations are called fibrillatory (f) waves. The rapid atrial impulses result in a quivering, ineffective motion of the atria, resulting in loss of the "atrial kick."

The AV node normally conducts supraventricular impulses at a rate no greater than 175 beats/min. Thus, most of the rapid irregular impulses in atrial fibrillation are *blocked* in the AV node. The impulses conducted to the ventricles produce QRS complexes that are usually narrow in configuration and occur at *irregularly irregular* intervals.

The ECG criteria of atrial fibrillation are as follows:

1. Irregular undulations of the baseline called fibrillation (f) waves. P waves are absent.
2. QRS complexes that are usually narrow in configuration and occur at irregularly irregular intervals.

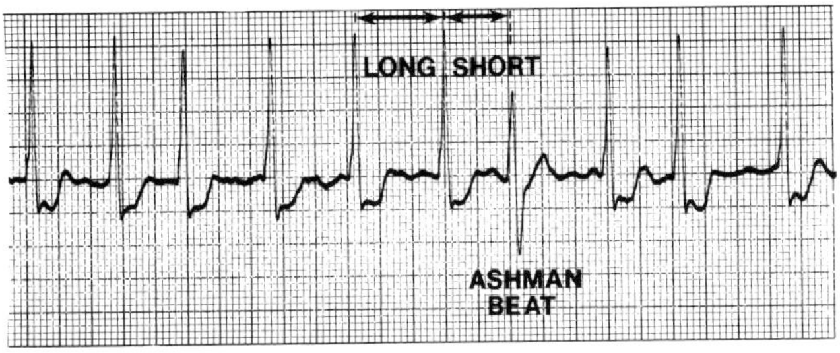

FIG 5–15.
Ashman beat. Note that the Ashman beat follows a *short* R-R cycle preceded by a *long* R-R cycle during atrial fibrillation. The early wide QRS complex *(Ashman beat)* at the end of the *short* cycle results from aberrant ventricular conduction. This example also demonstrates marked ST depression caused by subendocardial ischemia and/or "Dig. effect."

ASHMAN BEAT IN ATRIAL FIBRILLATION

If the ventricular rate is rapid during atrial fibrillation, the ventricles may be partially refractory to succeding impulses because they have not had time to fully repolarize. This results in aberrant ventricular conduction. Importantly, when a R-R interval (R-R cycle) is long and the next impulse is conducted early (short R-R interval), the QRS configuration of the early impulse will widen and become slurred because of aberrant ventricular conduction. This early wide QRS complex is known as the *Ashman beat* (see Fig 9–19,*B*).

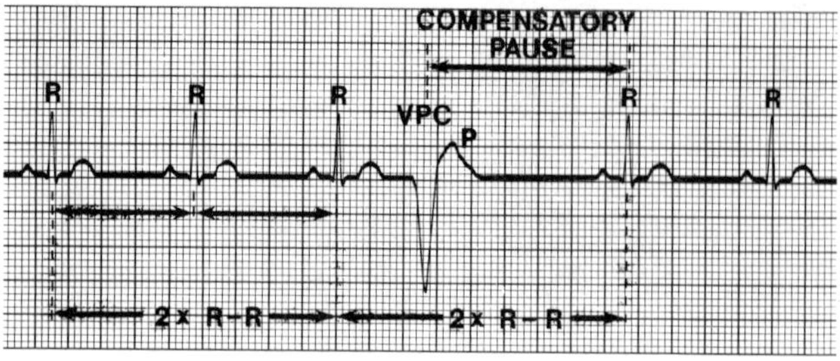

FIG 5–16.
Ventricular premature contraction *(VPC).* A nonconducted P wave *(P)* is seen in the *T* wave of the *VPC.* The *compensatory pause* is the interval between the *VPC* and next normally conducted sinus beat. The *compensatory pause* is confirmed by measuring the distance between the two normally conducted sinus beats that surround the *VPC.* This measured interval should equal twice the normal R-R interval *(2 × R-R).*

VENTRICULAR PREMATURE CONTRACTION

Ventricular premature contraction (VPC) is an abnormal QRS complex that originates from an ectopic focus *in the ventricles.* Depolarization from this ectopic focus proceeds slowly and abnormally (muscle cell to muscle cell) through the ventricles, producing a wide, bizarre QRS complex. The abnormal ventricular depolarization results in abnormal ventricular repolarization. That is, repolarization represented by the ST segment and T wave is usually opposite in direction to the main deflection of the QRS complex in a VPC. Additionally, because the impulse originates in the ventricles, there is not a sinus P wave preceding the QRS complex.

A VPC that interrupts normal sinus rhythm usually produces a long pause, termed *compensatory pause,* between the VPC and the next normally conducted sinus beat. The mechanism of the compensatory pause is that the *first* sinus impulse (P wave) following the VPC is blocked and unable to depolarize the ventricles. Usually the P wave representing this nonconducted sinus impulse can be seen in the T wave of the VPC (see figure). The ventricles are refractory to conduction from this sinus impulse. The succeeding, *second,* sinus impulse is conducted normally.

The compensatory pause denotes the time interval between the VPC and the next normally conducted sinus impulse. The compensatory pause is confirmed by measuring the distance between the two normally conducted sinus beats surrounding the VPC. This distance should be two times the baseline R-R interval.

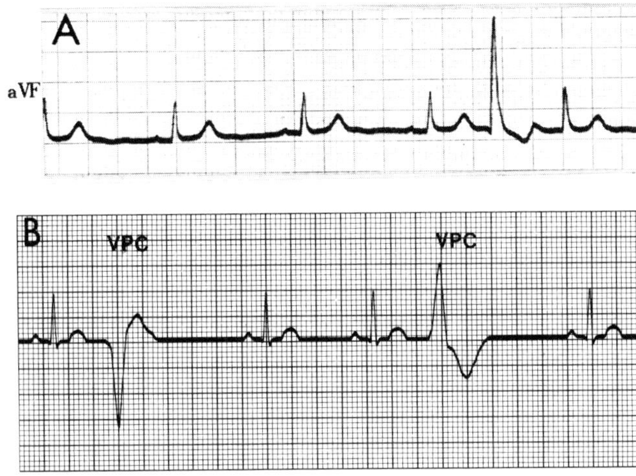

FIG 5–17.
A, interpolated VPC. **B,** multiform VPCs.

VPC PATTERNS

INTERPOLATED VPC.—This VPC occurs between two normal sinus beats *without* a compensatory pause. Note that the P-R interval of the sinus beat following the interpolated VPC is slightly longer than the normal P-R interval. This results from "concealed" retrograde conduction in the AV junction (see reference text).

MULTIFORM VPCs.—These VPCs display varying QRS configurations *in the same ECG lead.* The VPCs either originate from different foci in the ventricles or follow different pathways of conduction from a single ventricular focus. *Uniform* or *unifocal VPCs* are similar in configuration and originate from a single ventricular focus.

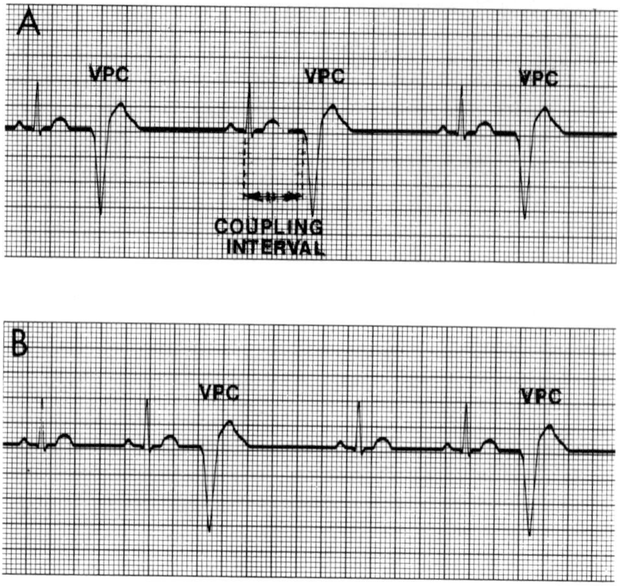

FIG 5–18.
A, bigeminy. **B,** trigeminy.

VPC PATTERNS

BIGEMINY.—In this pattern, each VPC alternates with a normal beat repeatedly. The VPC is coupled or associated with the preceding beat by a fixed *coupling interval.*

TRIGEMINY.—In this pattern, the VPC alternates with two normal beats repeatedly, or a normal beat alternates with two VPCs repeatedly.

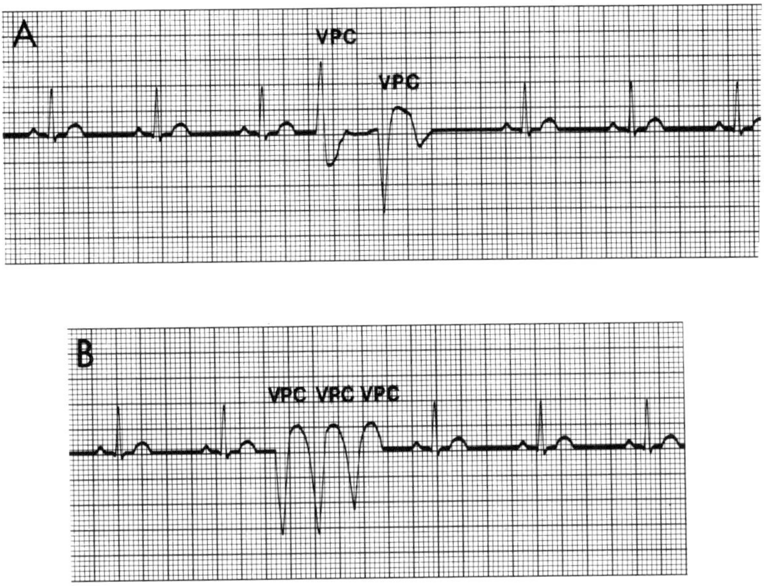

FIG 5–19.
A, couplet. **B,** triplet.

VPC PATTERNS

COUPLET.—A couplet is two VPCs in a row. The figure shows two multiform VPCs in a row.

TRIPLET.—A triplet is three VPCs in a row. Arbitrarily, three or more VPCs in a row is termed ventricular tachycardia.

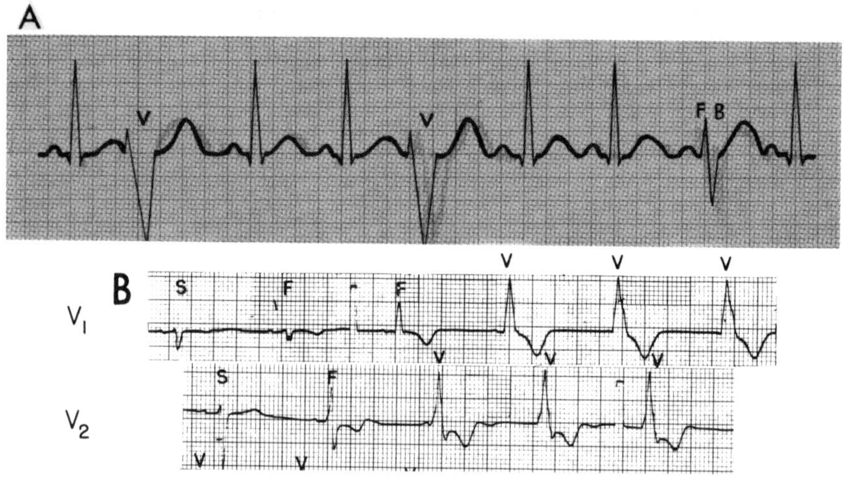

FIG 5–20.
A, ventricular parasystole. *V,* ventricular parasystole beats; *FB,* fusion beat. **B,** onset of accelerated idioventricular rhythm with fusion *(F)* beats. Note preceding P wave and mixed QRS configuration of the fusion beats compared to the sinus *(S)* and idioventricular *(V)* beats.

VPC PATTERNS

VENTRICULAR PARASYSTOLE.—This special type of rhythm involves two independent competing pacemakers: (1) the basic underlying rhythm and (2) an ectopic ventricular rhythm. The VPCs occur at regular, fixed intervals or multiples of the fixed intervals independent of the underlying rhythm. Criteria for ventricular parasystole include (1) distance between two parasystolic VPCs being a multiple of the shortest R-R interval between two parasystolic beats, (2) varying coupling intervals between VPCs and normal beats, (3) occasional fusion (Dressler) beats, and (4) unchanged QRS configuration of the parasystolic VPCs. In this figure, the two competing rhythms are normal sinus rhythm, rate of 75 beats/min and a slow ventricular parasystolic rhythm (26 beats/min). Note the varying coupling intervals. The third ventricular beat is a fusion beat *(FB)* with a P wave preceding the fusion beats.

FUSION (DRESSLER) BEAT.—This occurs when a supraventricular impulse conducts to the ventricles at approximately the same time that a ventricular ectopic impulse occurs. The two impulses fuse into one beat. In *B*, the fusion beats *(F)* represent the fusion of a sinus and an idioventricular beat. It is wider than the sinus conducted beat *(S)*, but narrower than the idioventricular beats *(V)*. The FB display various QRS configurations.

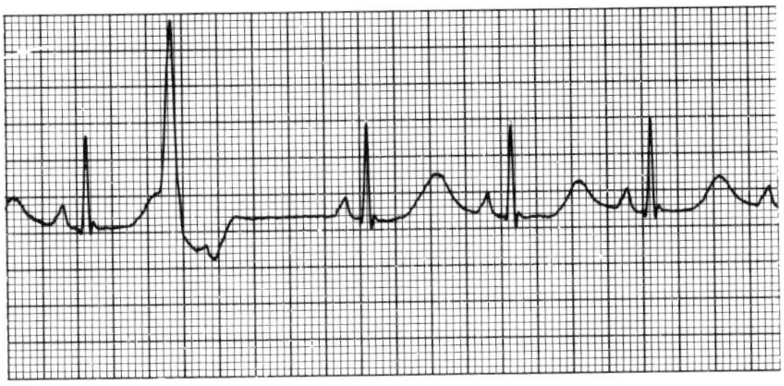

FIG 5–21.
R-on-T phenomenon. The R wave of the VPC occurs on or near the peak of the T wave.

VPC PATTERNS

R-ON-T PHENOMENON.—The VPC occurs on or near the peak of the previous T wave. This is the *vulnerable period* during ventricular repolarization and may predispose to ventricular tachycardia or ventricular fibrillation.

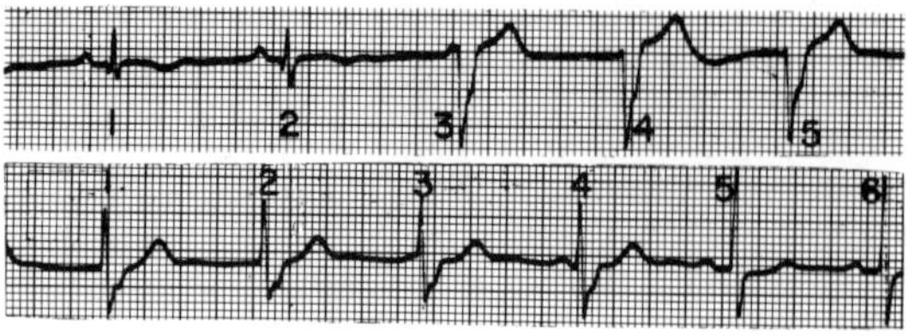

FIG 5–22.
Accelerated idioventricular rhythm. Note that the first beats (*1* and *2*) in lead I are preceded by P waves, indicating sinus-initiated beats. The QRS in beat *2* shows a slight variation (deeper S wave), indicating that it is a fusion beat. The succeeding beats *(3, 4, 5)* are idioventricular beats at a rate of 68 beats/min, which is faster than the usual idioventricular rate of 15 to 40 beats/min. In lead V_5, beats 1, 2, and 3 are not preceded by P waves and are idioventricular in origin. Starting with beat 4, P waves precede the QRS complexes, and the fifth and sixth complexes indicate a return to sinus rhythm.

ACCELERATED IDIOVENTRICULAR RHYTHM

Accelerated idioventricular rhythm is an enhanced ectopic ventricular rhythm whereby the pacemaker site in the ventricles fires at a rate of 40–100 beat/min (faster than the intrinsic ventricular pacemaker rate of 15–40 beats/min). It resembles ventricular tachycardia, with wide QRS complexes, AV dissociation, and occasional fusion beats, except that the rate is less than 100 beats/min. Accelerated idioventricular rhythm is usually characterized by runs of wide QRS complexes at a rate slightly faster than the sinus rate, and it sometimes alternates with periods of sinus rhythm. Ventricular fusion beats (see Fig 5–20) may herald the onset and termination of the rhythm (see above figure).

Accelerated idioventricular rhythm is most commonly seen within the first 48 to 72 hours of acute myocardial infarction and frequently after successful reperfusion during acute myocardial infarction (following thrombolysis or angioplasty). It is usually thought to be a benign arrhythmia which is transient. However, if cardiac function is compromised, agents such as atropine, isoproterenol, or pacemaker may be used to increase the intrinsic heart rate. Antiarrhythmic agents may also be used to treat this relatively benign arrhythmia.

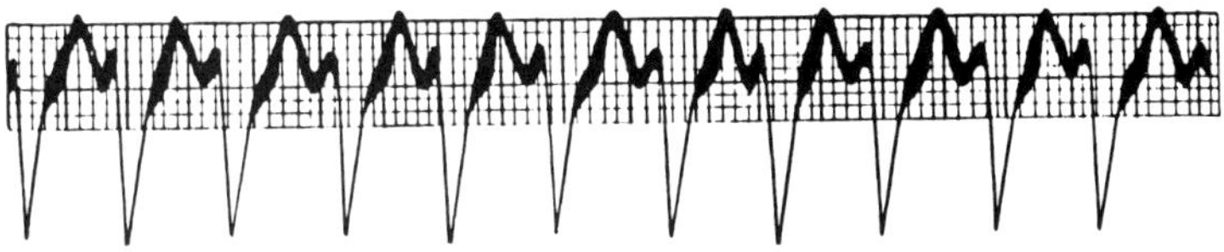

FIG 5–23.
Ventricular tachycardia. Wide QRS complex tachycardia at a rate of 175 beats/min.

VENTRICULAR TACHYCARDIA

Ventricular tachycardia is a ventricular rhythm of three or more VPCs in a row at a rate faster than 100 beats/min. Diagnostic ECG features of ventricular tachycardia include the following:

1. Wide (greater than 0.12 second), bizarre QRS complexes *in the absence of* preexisting bundle branch block, aberration, or preexcitation syndrome.
2. Rate faster than 100 beats/min.
3. P waves dissociated from QRS complexes (AV dissociation).
4. Occasional fusion (Dressler) beats.
5. Occasional sinus capture beats. A sinus capture beat occurs when a sinus impulse conducts to the ventricles (a P wave is followed by a normal-appearing QRS complex) during ventricular tachycardia.

Ventricular tachycardia may be classified as *sustained* or *nonsustained.* Sustained ventricular tachycardia may degenerate into ventricular fibrillation causing cardiac arrest. Nonsustained ventricular tachycardia consists of short salvos of three or more VPCs in a row. Treatment of ventricular tachycardia includes antiarrhythmic drugs, synchronized cardioversion (external or implantable), surgical techniques, and catheter ablation.

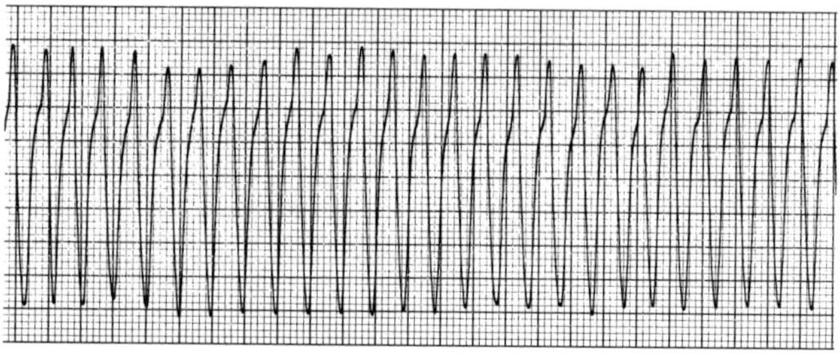

FIG 5–24.
Ventricular flutter. Observe the undulating regular QRS waves at a rate of 300 per minute without discernible ST and T deflections.

VENTRICULAR FLUTTER

Ventricular flutter is a ventricular rhythm characterized by undulating, regular QRS waves of large amplitude at a rate between 180 and 300 beats/min. The ST segments and T waves are not seen in ventricular flutter, whereas in ventricular tachycardia, these ST and T deflections can be seen. This rhythm is a precursor of ventricular fibrillation.

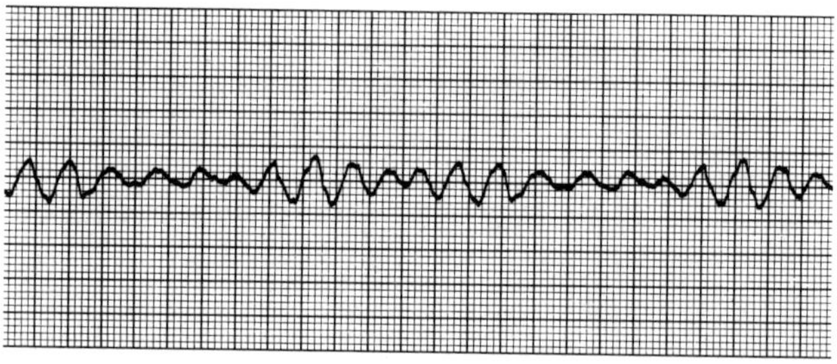

FIG 5–25.
Ventricular fibrillation. Note the irregular fibrillatory QRS waves. This represents no effective contractions of the ventricles, cardiac arrest.

VENTRICULAR FIBRILLATION

Ventricular fibrillation is a ventricular rhythm characterized by bizarre, irregularly irregular fibrillatory QRS waves up to a rate of 500 per minute. The ventricular fibrillation waves replace the P, QRS, and T waves. This rhythm represents completely disorganized electrical and mechanical activity in the heart (cardiac arrest), and if allowed to continue, results in death. Treatment includes cardiopulmonary resuscitation and electrical defibrillation.

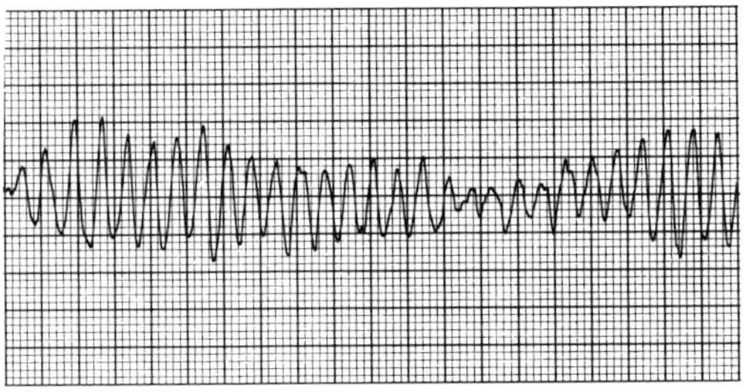

FIG 5–26.
Torsade de pointes. Observe the "twisting" of the peaks and troughs of the QRS complexes in relation to the baseline.

TORSADE DE POINTES

Torsade de pointes is a type of ventricular tachycardia originally described by Dessertenne as a "twisting of the points." As the figure shows, the peaks and troughs of the QRS complexes change their position in relation to the baseline. This rhythm either terminates spontaneously or degenerates into ventricular fibrillation.

The most common predisposing cause of torsade de pointes is prolongation of the Q-T interval, which may be acquired or congenital. Acquired mechanisms that prolong the Q-T interval include type I antiarrhythmic drugs (procainamide, quinidine, disopyramide), psychotropic drugs, electrolyte abnormalities (hypomagnesemia, hypokalemia, hypocalcemia), liquid protein diets, and other causes. Treatment includes removal of the predisposing cause as well as the use of lidocaine, bretylium, isoproterenol (Isuprel), phenytoin, β-adrenergic blockers, pacemaker, or electrical cardioversion. In patients who have recurrent episodes of torsade de pointes, left stellate ganglionectomy, as well as implantable cardioverter-defibrillators, have been utilized.

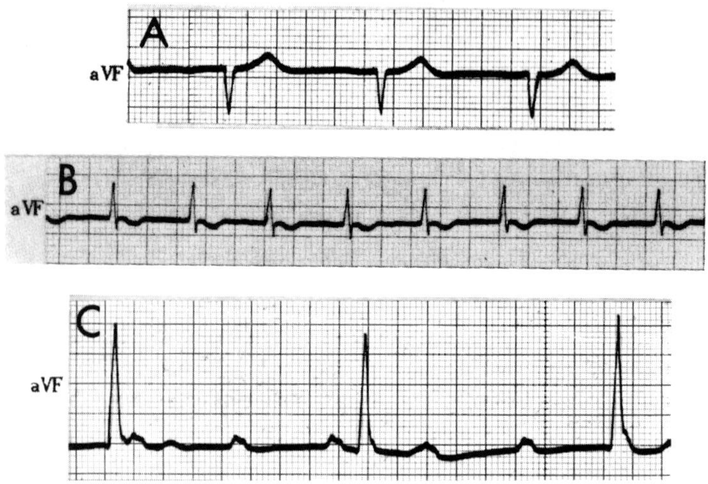

FIG 5–27.
Three mechanisms of AV dissociation. **A,** escape junctional rhythm at a rate of 58 beats/min in a patient with a slower sinus bradycardia. **B,** accelerated junctional rhythm at a rate of 115 beats/min, which usurps the underlying sinus rhythm. **C,** complete AV block. The atrial rate is 85 beats/min; the ventricular rate is 35 beats/min, and is entirely independent of the atria.

AV DISSOCIATION

Atrioventricular dissociation is a rhythm whereby the atria and ventricles are controlled by separate pacemakers. There are three primary mechanisms that may cause AV dissociation:

1. Primary pacemaker slows so that a subsidiary escape pacemaker site begins to fire. An example would be a sinus bradycardia at a rate of 40 beats/min with a subsidiary junctional escape pacemaker firing faster at a rate of 58 beats/min (Fig 5–27,*A*).

2. Primary pacemaker continues normally while a lower, enhanced subsidiary pacemaker (junctional or ventricular) fires faster. Examples are accelerated junctional rhythm or ventricular tachycardia in which the ventricles fire faster than the normal sinus rate (Fig 5–27,*B*).

3. Complete AV block occurs. An example is third-degree AV block (Fig 5–27,*C*).

4. In each of these conditions, there is dissocation between atrial and ventricular activation. Note that AV dissociation is only a descriptive term that provides no information regarding the primary cause of the arrhythmia.

PEARLS

1. The Lewis lead (see p. 45) is used to identify difficult-to-find P waves. This lead is a modification of standard ECG lead I. The right arm electrode is placed in the *second right* intercostal space, and the left arm electrode is placed in the *fourth right* intercostal space. These electrodes are in close proximity to the atria so that P waves may be more readily visualized. Utilize all 12 leads to identify P waves and QRS contours.

2. The most common cause of a pause in the ECG is a blocked APC, which results in an absent QRS complex. Observe preceding T wave closely for evidence of the APC.

3. An APC usually *activates* and *resets* the SA node. This results in a pause that is not compensatory between the APC and next SA-conducted beat.

4. An APC is usually recognized by a *premature* normal-appearing QRS complex that is preceded by a bizarre or inverted P wave.

5. The early P wave of an APC frequently distorts the preceding T wave.

6. While MAT may resemble atrial fibrillation, a careful search for P waves will help differentiate them. Look in *all* 12 leads for P waves.

7. In a resting ECG with a ventricular rate of 150 beats/min, think of atrial flutter with 2:1 block. The interpreter must search for flutter waves in leads II, III, aVF, V_1, V_2. Vagal maneuvers may slow the ventricular response so that the flutter waves become more visible.

8. The atrial flutter rate slows (250 beats/min or less) and the flutter waves widen in patients taking the type I antiarrhythmic agent quinidine.

9. A VPC that originates from the right ventricle resembles the configuration of a left bundle branch block (LBBB) pattern. Conversely, a VPC that originates from the left ventricle resembles the configuration of a right bundle branch block pattern.

6 / Heart Block

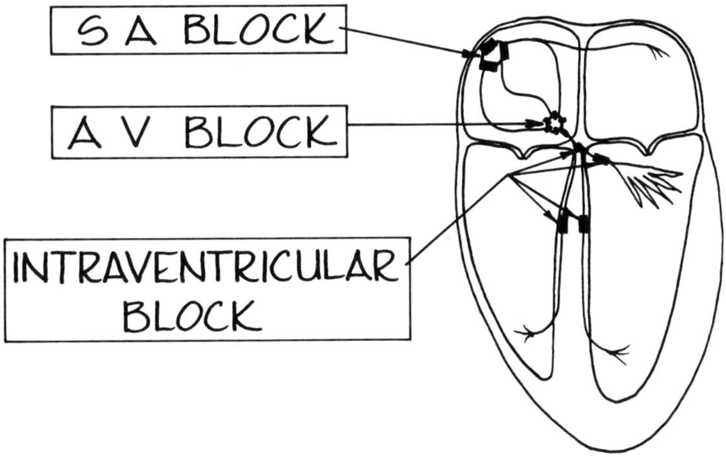

FIG 6–1.
Heart block diagrammatically depicted as *solid bars.* Heart block may occur in the SA node *(SA block),* AV node *(AV block),* or in the ventricles *(intraventricular block).*

Heart block indicates a delay or obstruction in the conduction of the electrical impulses in the heart. The block may occur anywhere in the specialized conducting system or in the muscle of the heart. In the ECG, heart block may be divided anatomically into the following:

1. SA block (sinoatrial block)
2. AV block (atrioventricular block)
3. Intraventricular block (bundle branch block and fascicular block)

There are numerous causes of heart block, which include drugs, ischemia, injury, infarction, aging, and hypertrophy.

SA BLOCK

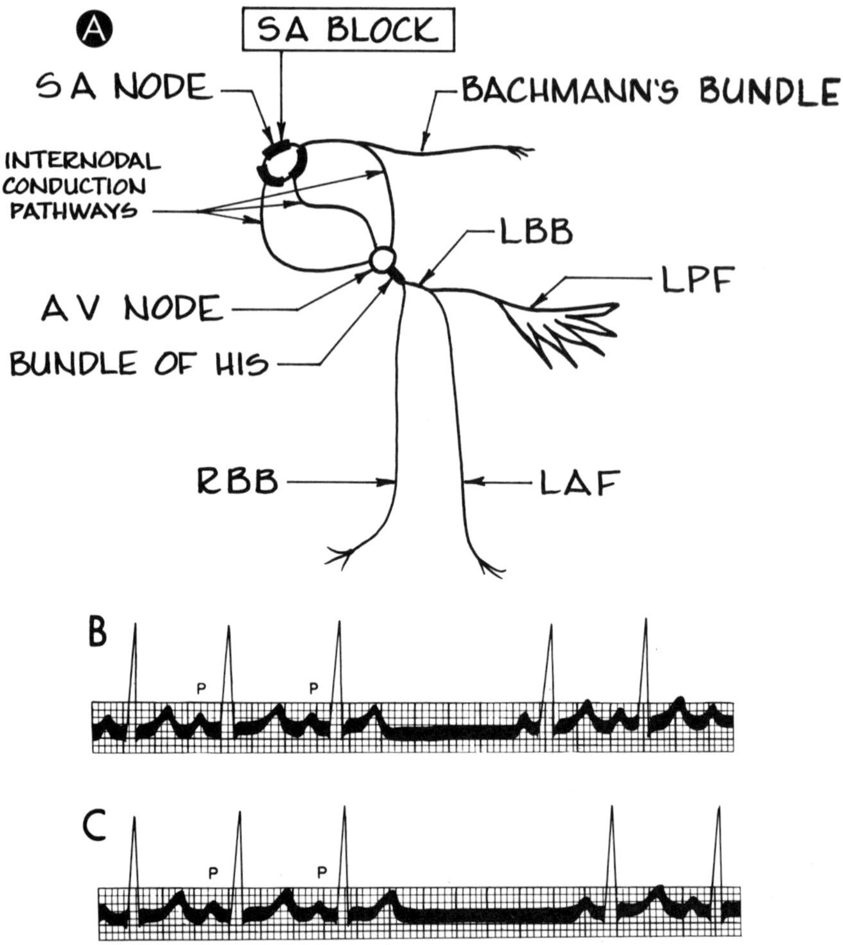

FIG 6–2.
A, *SA* (sinoatrial) *block* located around the *SA node.* Specialized conducting system. *AV* (atrioventricular) node; *RBB,* right bundle branch; *LBB,* left bundle branch; *LAF,* left anterior fascicle; *LPF,* left posterior fascicle. **B,** SA block. There is absence of the P-QRS-T complex, and the interval between sinus beats surrounding the SA block is a multiple of the previous P-P interval. **C,** sinus pause. The P-P interval surrounding the pause is *not* a multiple of the previous P-P intervals.

SA BLOCK

SA Block vs. Sinus Pause

SA *block* indicates impaired conduction of electrical impulses from the SA node into the atria. Remember that the P wave represents depolarization of the atrial muscle cells. In SA block, impaired conduction from the SA node results in no depolarization of the atria and absence of the entire P-QRS-T complex. The hallmark of SA block is a missing P wave and its QRS complex. Importantly, the duration of the interval between the two normal beats is usually a multiple of the previous P-P intervals.

SA *block* should be differentiated from *sinus pause* (also termed sinus arrest or sinus standstill), which occurs when there is failure to generate a sinus impulse from the SA node. During sinus pause, there is absence of an entire heart beat (no P wave or QRS complex). However, the duration of the pause is usually *not* a multiple of the previous P-P intervals.

Factors that may cause SA block or sinus pause include the following:

1. Increased vagal tone
2. Drugs
3. Inferior myocardial infarction
4. Degeneration from aging

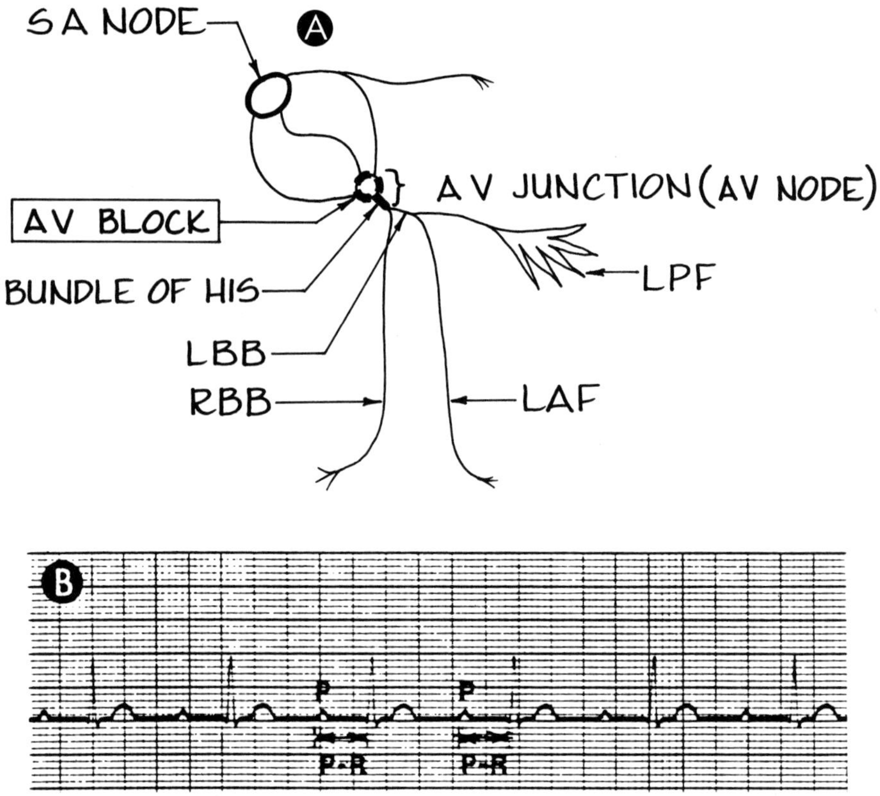

FIG 6–3.
A, first degree *AV block* is caused by a conduction delay in the *AV junction.* **B,** sinus rhythm, first-degree AV block. The *P-R* interval is prolonged to 0.32 second.

AV BLOCK

First Degree

The occurrence of *AV block* indicates a delay or obstruction in the transmission of impulses from the atria to the ventricles. The block is located in the AV junction. There are three divisions of severity in AV block: first, second, and third degree.

First-degree AV block is characterized by a partial block in the AV node (AV junction), which causes *prolongation* of the P-R interval to greater than 0.20 second (normal P-R interval is 0.12–0.20 second). All of the P waves are followed by QRS complexes. However, because of the conduction delay in the AV junction, the P-R interval is lengthened.

Causes of first-degree AV block are similar to those of SA block and include drugs (especially digoxin), increased vagal tone, aging, and acute inferior myocardial infarction.

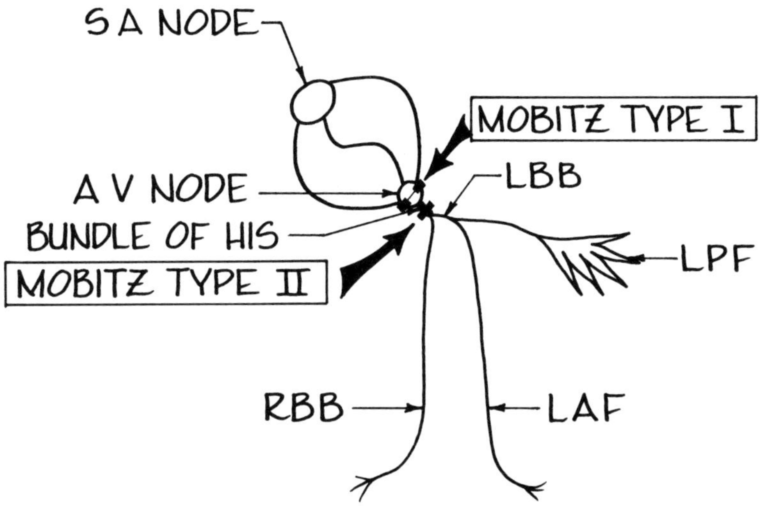

FIG 6–4.
Second-degree AV block. *Mobitz type I* (Wenckebach) block is located in the higher area of the AV junction. *Mobitz type II* block is usually located in the lower area of the AV junction, in the *bundle of His,* or lower; and it is a more serious arrhythmia than Mobitz type I block.

AV BLOCK

Second Degree

In *second-degree AV block,* some but not all atrial impulses are totally blocked in the AV node and fail to conduct to the ventricles so that some P waves are not followed by QRS complexes. Second-degree AV block is divided into two types: *Mobitz Type I (Wenckebach)* and *Mobitz Type II.*

Anatomically, Mobitz type I second-degree AV block is usually located in the higher areas of the AV junction. Mobitz type II second-degree AV block is usually located in the lower area of the AV junction, in the area of the bundle of His or lower. Mobitz type II AV block is usually but not always associated with a *wide QRS complex* because of an associated *intraventricular conduction block* (right bundle branch block [RBBB], left bundle branch block [LBBB], left anterior fascicular block [LAFB], left posterior fascicular block [LPFB], or combination of these blocks). Because of its lower location, Mobitz type II second-degree AV block is considered a more serious rhythm disturbance than Mobitz type I.

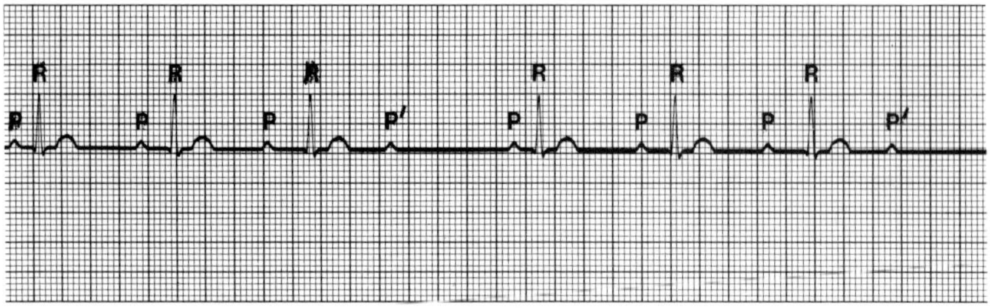

FIG 6–5.
Mobitz I (Wenckebach) second-degree AV block. The P-R intervals gradually lengthen, the P-P intervals remain equal, and the R-R intervals gradually shorten until a nonconducted beat *(P')* occurs. Note the pattern of grouped beating.

SECOND-DEGREE AV BLOCK

Mobitz Type I (Wenckebach)

Second-degree AV block, Mobitz type I, is customarily referred to as *Wenckebach* block. It is characterized by a progressive increase in the length of successive P-R intervals until a P wave finally fails to conduct to the ventricles. This cycle usually repeats itself, causing the beats to appear grouped, *grouped beating* (see figure). The ECG criteria for second-degree AV block, Mobitz type I (Wenckebach) are as follows:

1. Grouped beating.
2. Progressive lengthening of P-R interval until a P wave is completely blocked, resulting in an absent QRS complex.
3. Constant P-P intervals.
4. Progressive shortening of the R-R interval until the block occurs.
5. The longest R-R interval surrounding the dropped QRS complex is less than twice the shortest R-R interval (see reference text).

The basic mechanism of the Wenckebach phenomenon is that conduction through the AV junction progressively lengthens until it is totally blocked for one beat. Importantly, the P-R interval progressively lengthens, but it does so by decreasing increments. That is, the P-R interval progressively gets longer, but it gets longer by smaller and smaller increments with each beat. This causes the P-R interval to lengthen and the R-R interval to shorten until conduction is totally blocked. Then the cycle repeats itself. Common causes of Wenckebach or Mobitz type I second-degree AV block include drugs (digoxin) and acute inferior myocardial infarction.

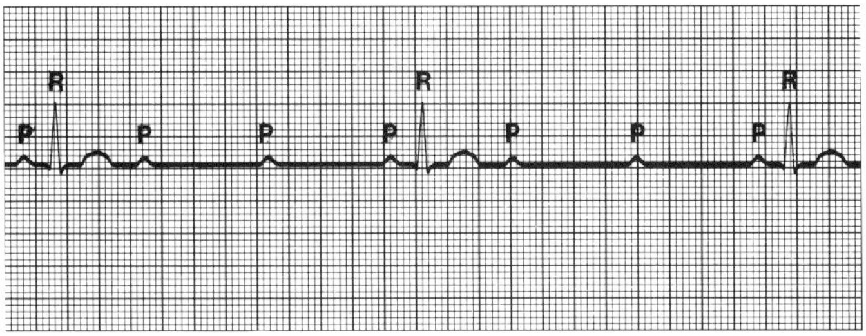

FIG 6–6.
Mobitz II second-degree AV block. There are three *P* waves for every QRS complex; this represents 3:1 AV block, high-degree AV block. Note that the P-R intervals of the conducted beats are constant.

SECOND-DEGREE AV BLOCK

Mobitz Type II

In second-degree AV block, *Mobitz type II,* a more serious type of AV block, an atrial impulse (P wave) suddenly fails to conduct to the ventricles. There is no prolongation of the P-R intervals prior to the blocked P wave. The ECG reveals P waves followed by QRS complexes and sudden intermittent blocked P waves that are not followed by QRS complexes. The P-P intervals are constant (including the nonconducted P wave), and the P-R intervals of normally conducted beats maintain a constant length.

The relation between the number of atrial impulses (P waves) to the number of impulses that reach the ventricles (QRS complexes) is called the *A:V ratio.* The A:V ratio (P waves: QRS complexes) is usually 2:1, 3:2, 4:3, etc. High-degree or advanced AV block occurs when the A:V ratio is 3:1 (three P waves to every QRS complex) or greater (4:1, 5:1, etc.). In high-degree AV block, escape rhythms frequently occur.

In Mobitz type II block, the QRS is usually wide because the block is low in the AV junction or in the bundle of His or lower in the specialized conducting system resulting in an intraventricular block. In Mobitz type I AV block, the QRS is usually narrow because of the higher location (upper part of AV junction) and subsequent normal intraventricular conduction.

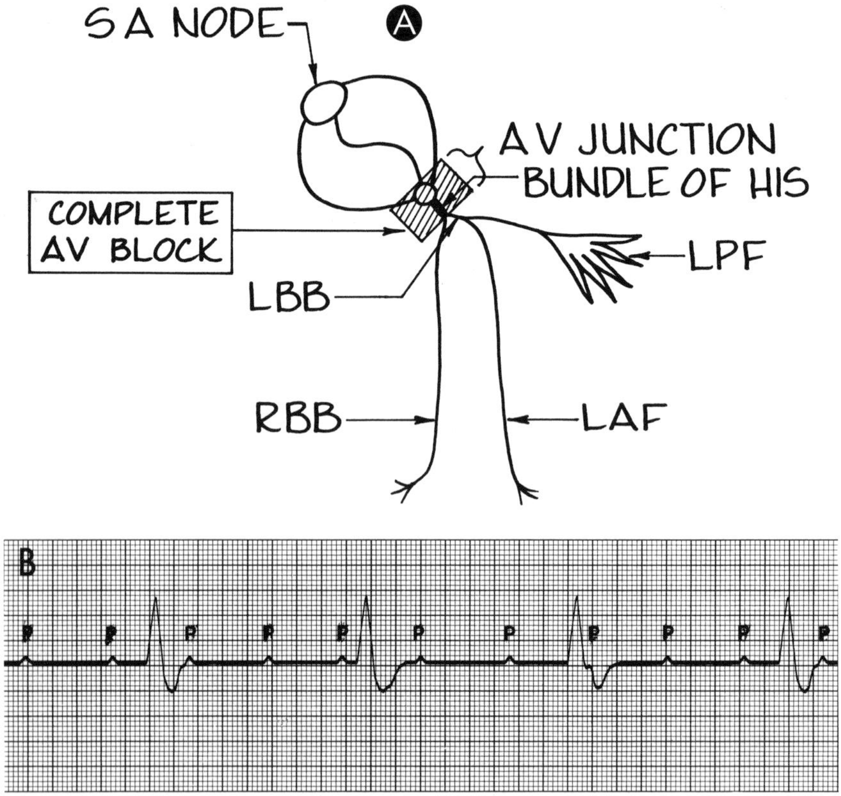

FIG 6–7.
A, *complete AV block* may be located in the *AV junction* or in the *bundle of His.* **B,** complete AV block. The atria (*P* waves) beat faster (rate of 80 beats/min) and independently of the ventricles (ventricular escape rate 35 beats/min).

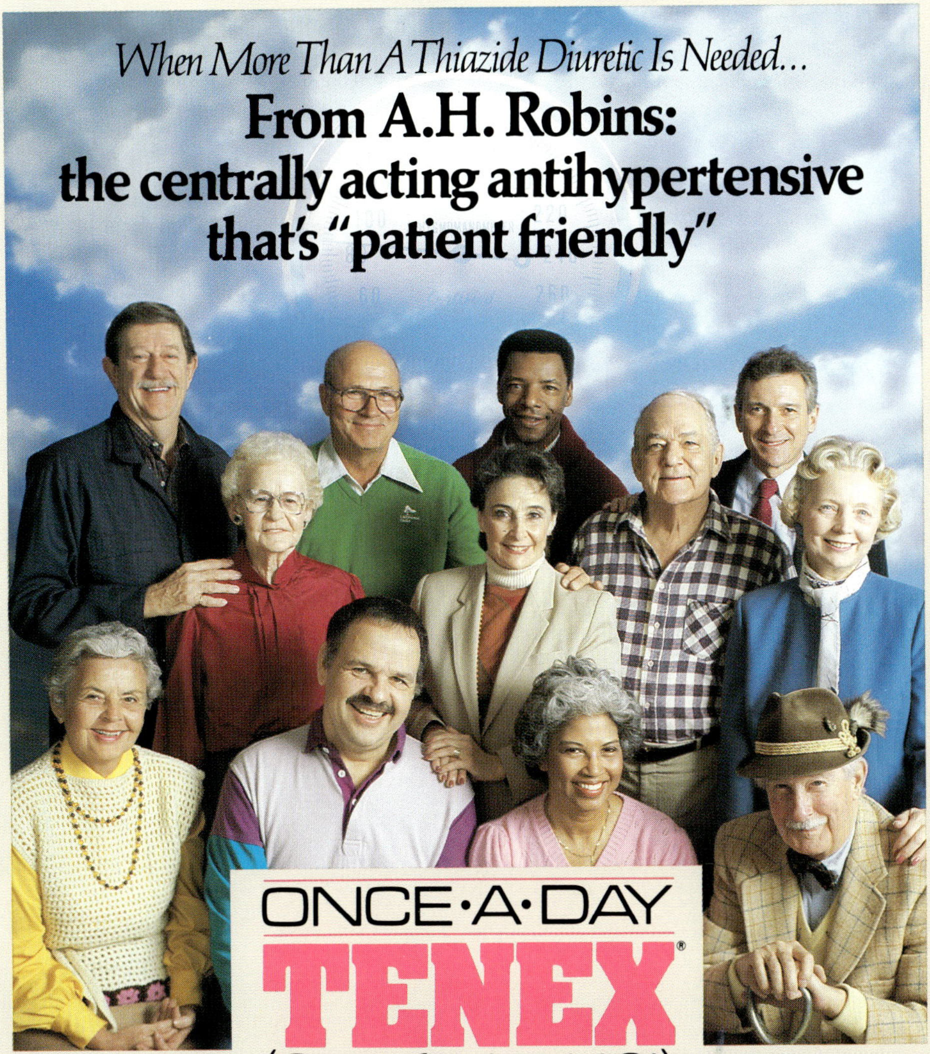

(Guanfacine HCl)

- A side effect profile at 1 mg/day comparable to placebo
  Fewer patient complaints
- 1 mg a day — optimal dosage for most patients
  Most patients will not require dose titration
- Once a day, for 24-hour control
  Convenience and compliance
- Suitable for a wide range of patients

A·H·ROBINS
Pharmaceutical Division, Richmond, Virginia 23261-6609

Please see prescribing information on the following page.

TENEX®

(Guanfacine HCl)

The following is a brief summary only. Before prescribing, see complete prescribing information in Tenex product labeling.

Contraindications: Tenex is contraindicated in patients with known hypersensitivity to guanfacine hydrochloride.

Precautions: *General.* Like other antihypertensive agents, Tenex (guanfacine hydrochloride) should be used with caution in patients with severe coronary insufficiency, recent myocardial infarction, cerebrovascular disease or chronic renal or hepatic failure.

Sedation. Tenex, like other orally active central alpha-2 adrenergic agonists, causes sedation or drowsiness, especially when beginning therapy. These symptoms are dose-related (see Adverse Reactions). When Tenex is used with other centrally active depressants (such as phenothiazines, barbiturates, or benzodiazepines), the potential for additive sedative effects should be considered.

Rebound. Abrupt cessation of therapy with orally active central alpha-2 adrenergic agonists may be associated with increases (from depressed on-therapy levels) in plasma and urinary catecholamines, symptoms of "nervousness and anxiety" and, less commonly, increases in blood pressure to levels significantly greater than those prior to therapy.

Information for Patients. Patients who receive Tenex should be advised to exercise caution when operating dangerous machinery or driving motor vehicles until it is determined that they do not become drowsy or dizzy from the medication. Patients should be warned that their tolerance for alcohol and other CNS depressants may be diminished. Patients should be advised not to discontinue therapy abruptly.

Laboratory Tests. In clinical trials, no clinically relevant laboratory test abnormalities were identified as causally related to drug during short-term treatment with Tenex (guanfacine hydrochloride).

Drug Interactions. No specific adverse drug interactions have been identified, but the potential for increased sedation when Tenex is given with other CNS-depressant drugs should be appreciated.

Anticoagulants. Ten patients who were stabilized on oral anticoagulants were given guanfacine, 1–2 mg/day, for 4 weeks. No changes were observed in the degree of anticoagulation.

In several well-controlled studies, guanfacine was administered together with diuretics with no drug interactions reported. In the long-term safety studies, Tenex was given concomitantly with many drugs without evidence of any interactions. The principal drugs given (number of patients in parentheses) were: cardiac glycosides (115), sedatives and hypnotics (103), coronary vasodilators (52), oral hypoglycemics (45), cough and cold preparations (45), NSAIDs (38), antihyperlipidemics (29), antigout drugs (24), oral contraceptives (18), bronchodilators (13), insulin (10), and beta blockers (10).

Drug/Laboratory Test Interactions. No laboratory test abnormalities related to the use of Tenex (guanfacine hydrochloride) have been identified.

Carcinogenesis, Mutagenesis, Impairment of Fertility. No carcinogenic effect was observed in studies of 78 weeks in mice at doses more than 150 times the maximum recommended human dose and 102 weeks in rats at doses more than 100 times the maximum recommended human dose. In a variety of test models guanfacine was not mutagenic.

No adverse effects were observed in fertility studies in male and female rats.

Pregnancy Category B. Administration of guanfacine to rats at 70 times the maximum recommended human dose and rabbits at 20 times the maximum recommended human dose resulted in no evidence of impaired fertility or harm to the fetus. Higher doses (100 and 200 times the maximum recommended human dose in rabbits and rats respectively) were associated with reduced fetal survival and maternal toxicity. Rat experiments have shown that guanfacine crosses the placenta.

There are, however, no adequate and well-controlled studies in pregnant women. Because animal reproduction studies are not always predictive of human response, this drug should be used during pregnancy only if clearly needed.

Labor and Delivery. Tenex (guanfacine hydrochloride) is not recommended in the treatment of acute hypertension associated with toxemia of pregnancy. There is no information available on the effects of guanfacine on the course of labor and delivery.

Nursing Mothers. It is not known whether Tenex (guanfacine hydrochloride) is excreted in human milk. Because many drugs are excreted in human milk, caution should be exercised when Tenex is administered to a nursing woman. Experiments with rats have shown that guanfacine is excreted in the milk.

Pediatric Use. Safety and effectiveness in children under 12 years of age have not been demonstrated. Therefore, the use of Tenex in this age group is not recommended.

Adverse Reactions: Adverse reactions noted with Tenex (guanfacine hydrochloride) are similar to those of other drugs of the central α-2 adrenoreceptor agonist class: dry mouth, sedation (somnolence), weakness (asthenia), dizziness, constipation, and impotence. While the reactions are common, most are mild and tend to disappear on continued dosing.

In a 12-week placebo-controlled, dose-response study the frequency of the most commonly observed adverse reactions showed a clear dose relationship from 0.5 to 3 mg, as follows:

Adverse Reaction	Assigned Treatment Group				
	Placebo	0.5 mg	1.0 mg	2.0 mg	3.0 mg
n =	73	72	72	72	72
Dry Mouth	5 (7%)	4 (5%)	6 (8%)	8 (11%)	20 (28%)
Somnolence	1 (1%)	3 (4%)	0 (0%)	1 (1%)	10 (14%)
Asthenia	0 (0%)	2 (3%)	0 (0%)	2 (2%)	7 (10%)
Dizziness	2 (2%)	1 (1%)	3 (4%)	6 (8%)	3 (4%)
Headache	3 (4%)	4 (3%)	3 (4%)	1 (1%)	2 (2%)
Impotence	1 (1%)	1 (1%)	0 (0%)	1 (1%)	3 (4%)
Constipation	0 (0%)	0 (0%)	0 (0%)	1 (1%)	1 (1%)
Fatigue	3 (3%)	2 (3%)	2 (3%)	5 (6%)	3 (4%)

There were 41 premature terminations because of adverse reactions in this study. The percent of patients who terminated and the dose at which they terminated were as follows:

Dose:	Placebo	0.5 mg	1 mg	2 mg	3 mg
Terminated:	6.9%	4.2%	3.2%	6.9%	8.3%

Reasons for dropouts among patients who received guanfacine were: somnolence, headache, weakness, dry mouth, dizziness, impotence, insomnia, constipation, syncope, urinary incontinence, conjunctivitis, paresthesia, and dermatitis.

In a second placebo-controlled study in which the dose could be adjusted upward to 3 mg per day in 1-mg increments at 3-week intervals, i.e., a setting more similar to ordinary clinical use, the most commonly recorded reactions were: dry mouth 47%, constipation 16%, fatigue 12%, somnolence 10%, asthenia 6%, dizziness 6%, headache 4%, and insomnia 4%.

Reasons for dropouts among patients who received guanfacine were: somnolence, dry mouth, dizziness, impotence, constipation, confusion, depression, and palpitations.

In the clonidine/guanfacine comparison described in Clinical Pharmacology, the most common adverse reactions noted were:

	Guanfacine (n = 279)	Clonidine (n = 278)
Dry mouth	30%	37%
Somnolence	21%	35%
Dizziness	11%	8%
Constipation	10%	5%
Fatigue	9%	8%
Headache	4%	4%
Insomnia	4%	3%

Adverse reactions occurring in 3% or less of patients in the three controlled trials were:

Cardiovascular—	bradycardia, palpitations, substernal pain
Gastrointestinal—	abdominal pain, diarrhea, dyspepsia, dysphagia, nausea
CNS—	amnesia, confusion, depression, insomnia, libido decrease
ENT disorders—	rhinitis, taste perversion, tinnitus
Eye disorders—	conjunctivitis, iritis, vision disturbance
Musculoskeletal—	leg cramps, hypokinesia
Respiratory—	dyspnea
Dermatologic—	dermatitis, pruritus, purpura, sweating
Urogenital—	testicular disorder, urinary incontinence
Other—	malaise, paresthesia, paresis

Adverse reaction reports tend to decrease over time. In an open-label trial of one year's duration, 580 hypertensive subjects were given guanfacine, titrated to achieve goal blood pressure, alone (51%), with diuretic (38%), with beta blocker (3%), with diuretic plus beta blocker (6%), or with diuretic plus vasodilator (2%). The mean daily dose of guanfacine reached was 4.7 mg.

Adverse Reaction	Incidence of adverse reactions at any time during the study	Incidence of adverse reactions at end of one year
	n = 580	n = 580
Dry mouth	60%	15%
Drowsiness	33%	6%
Dizziness	15%	1%
Constipation	14%	3%
Weakness	5%	1%
Headache	4%	0.2%
Insomnia	5%	0%

There were 52 (8.9%) dropouts due to adverse effects in this 1-year trial. The causes were: dry mouth (n = 20), weakness (n = 12), constipation (n = 7), somnolence (n = 3), nausea (n = 3), orthostatic hypotension (n = 2), insomnia (n = 1), rash (n = 1), nightmares (n = 1), headache (n = 1), and depression (n = 1).

Drug Abuse and Dependence: No reported abuse or dependence has been associated with the administration of Tenex (guanfacine hydrochloride).

A·H·ROBINS

Pharmaceutical Division
Richmond, Virginia 23261-6609

AV BLOCK

Third-Degree (Complete)

Third-degree AV block, complete heart block, denotes complete obstruction of impulse conduction from the atria to the ventricles. The atria (P waves) beat independently of the ventricles (QRS complexes) (see AV dissociation, Fig 5–27,*C*).

Because of the complete obstruction to conduction in the AV junction, a (lower) junctional or ventricular "escape" rhythm occurs. If the escape rhythm is junctional in origin (narrow QRS complexes), the ventricular rate is usually 40–60 beats/min. If the escape rhythm is ventricular in origin (wide QRS complexes), the rate is usually 15–40 beats/min.

In the presence of sinus rhythm and third-degree AV block, the P waves "march through" the independently beating QRS complexes. The P-P intervals usually remain constant, as do the R-R intervals. However, the atrial rate is usually faster than the ventricular rate.

Causes of third-degree AV block include drugs (digoxin), degeneration from aging, and acute myocardial infarction.

INTRAVENTRICULAR BLOCK

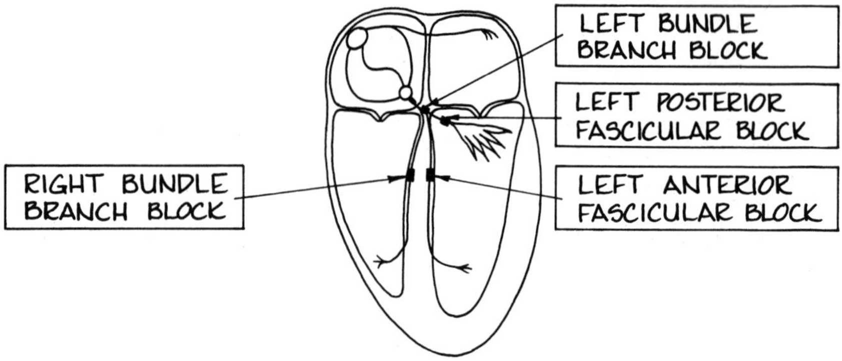

FIG 6–8.
Intraventricular block may occur in the right bundle branch (RBB), in the left bundle branch (LBB), in the left anterior fascicle (LAF), or left posterior fascicle (LPF).

INTRAVENTRICULAR BLOCK

Intraventricular block refers to impaired conduction in the *ventricular conducting system* below the bundle of His, which results in a wide QRS complex. The block may occur in the right bundle branch (RBB), left bundle branch (LBB), left anterior fascicle (LAF), or left posterior fascicle (LPF). Occasionally, the intraventricular block (wide QRS complex) may not be localized or identified. The wide QRS is then referred to as "nonspecific intraventricular conduction delay."

RIGHT BUNDLE BRANCH BLOCK

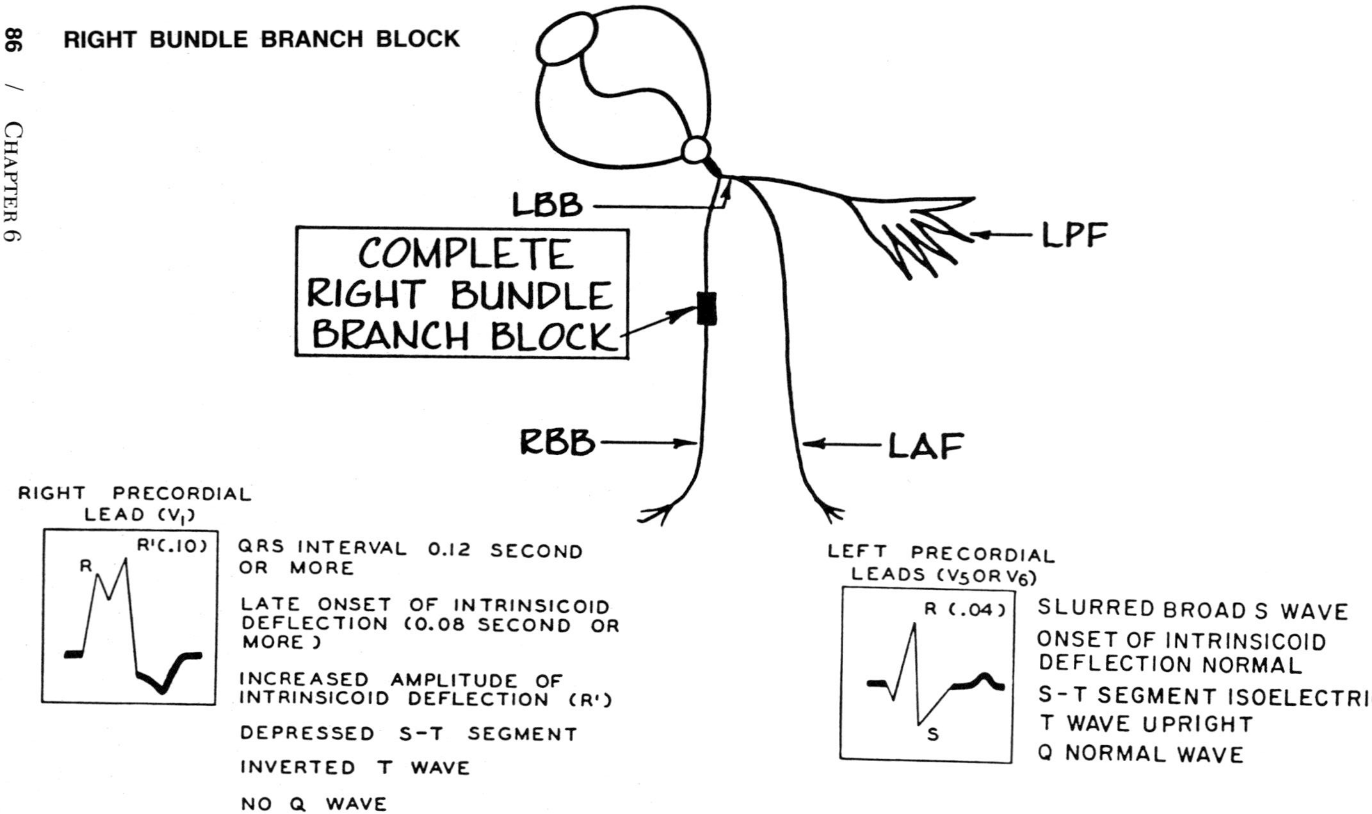

FIG 6–9.
Complete right bundle branch block. Right chest lead (V_1) and left chest leads (V_5, V_6). *LBB,* left bundle branch; *RBB,* right bundle branch; *LPF,* left posterior fascicle; LAF, left anterior fascicle.

RIGHT BUNDLE BRANCH BLOCK

In RBBB, the last portion of the heart to be activated is the right ventricle. The chest leads representing the right ventricle are leads V_1, V_2. *In RBBB, the late depolarization forces travel toward the right ventricle.* This causes the last part of the wide QRS complex to be positive (upright R′ wave) in lead V_1, and negative (downward S wave) in leads V_5, V_6.

Importantly, the RBBB prolongs the QRS complex to greater than 0.12 second.

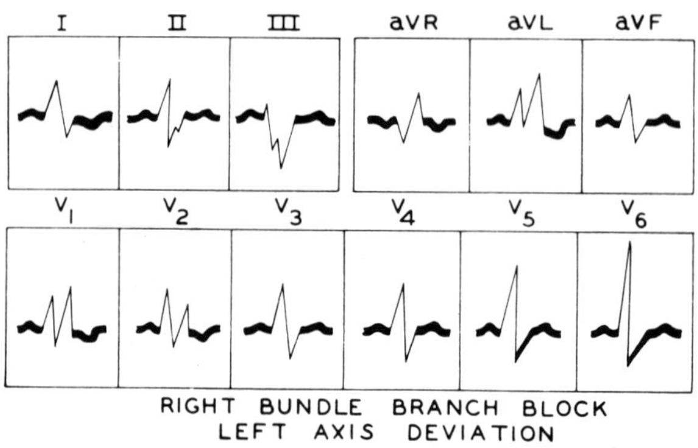

FIG 6–10.
Complete right bundle branch block. Note the QRS duration greater than 0.12 second; RSR′ in V_1, V_2; repolarization changes in V_1, V_2; deep S wave in V_5, V_6 (and I, aVL); and delayed onset of the intrinsicoid deflection in V_1, V_2.

CRITERIA FOR COMPLETE RBBB

The ECG criteria for *complete RBBB* are as follows:

1. QRS duration greater than 0.12 second.
2. RSR′ in the "right ventricular" leads V_1, V_2. The R′ represents late activation of the right ventricle as recorded in the "right ventricular" leads.
3. Wide or slurred S wave (negative deflection) in the "left ventricular" leads V_5, V_6 (also I, aVL). This represents late activation of the right ventricle as recorded in the "left ventricular" leads.
4. Ventricular repolarization changes (downsloping ST segment and inverted T wave—opposite direction to R′ wave) in leads V_1, V_2.
5. Late onset of intrinsicoid deflection (R peak time) in leads V_1, V_2 (greater than 0.04 second). This represents delayed onset of right ventricular activation.
6. Initial portion of the QRS complex in leads V_1, V_2 is positive. This represents the normal initial septal depolarization in RBBB. (See reference text.)

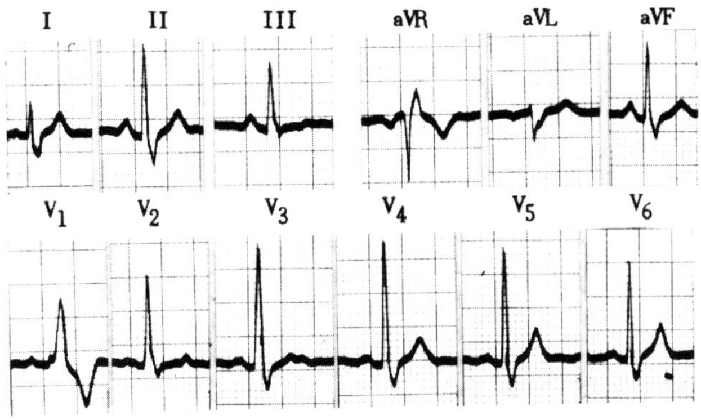

FIG 6–11.
Incomplete RBBB. Note the QRS duration between 0.10 and 0.12 second and the similar criteria for RBBB.

INCOMPLETE RBBB

The ECG criteria for *incomplete RBBB* include the following:

1. QRS duration between 0.10 and 0.12 second.
2. RSR′ in leads V_1 or V_2.
3. Broad S wave in leads V_5, V_6, (also I, aVL).
4. Late onset of intrinsicoid deflection (R peak time) in leads V_1 and V_2 (greater than 0.04 second).

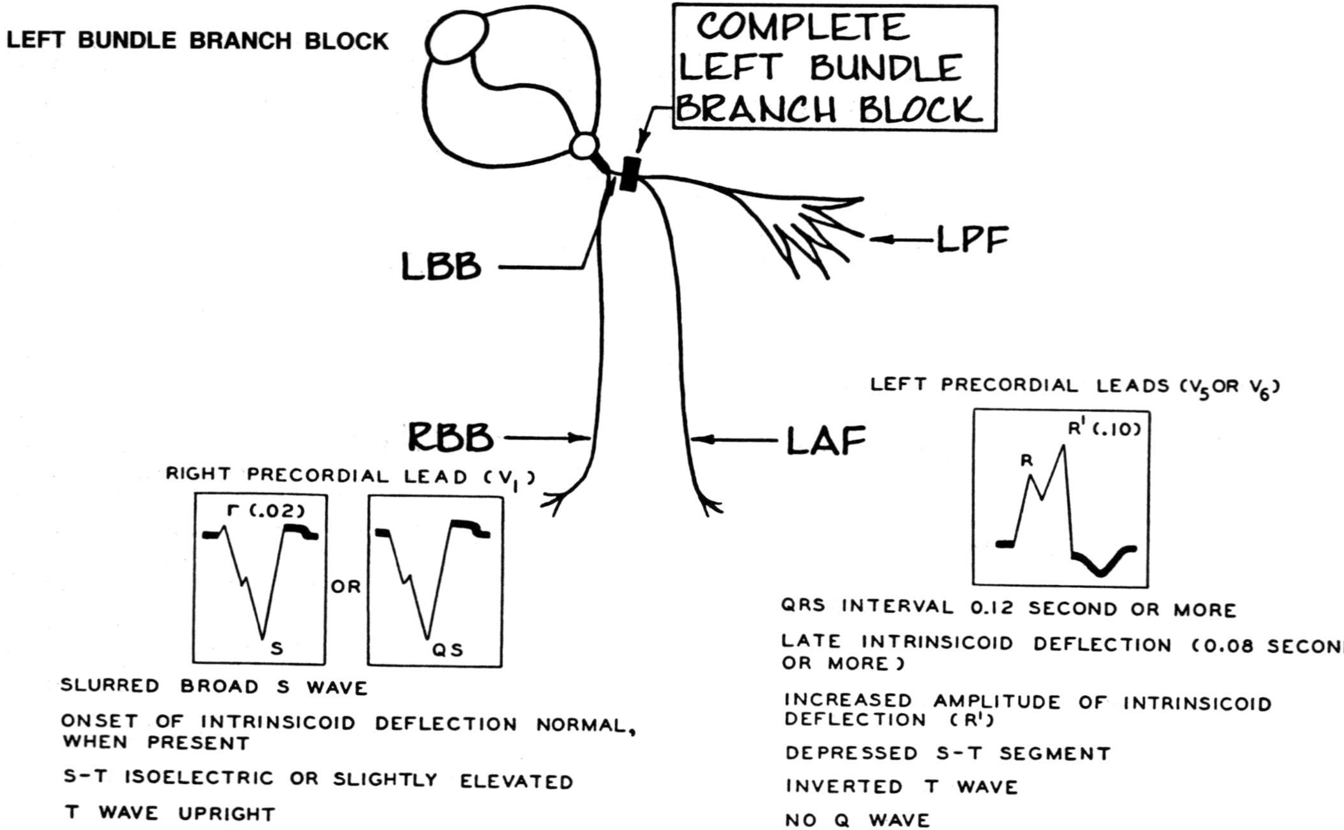

FIG 6–12.
Complete *left bundle branch block.* Right chest lead (V_1) and left chest leads (V_5, V_6). *LBB,* left bundle branch; *RBB,* right bundle branch; *LPF,* left posterior fascicle; *LAF,* left anterior fascicle.

LEFT BUNDLE BRANCH BLOCK

In LBBB, the last portion of the heart to be activated is the left ventricle. The chest leads representing the left ventricle are leads V_5, V_6. *In LBBB, the late depolarization forces travel toward the left ventricle.* This causes the last part of the wide QRS complex to be negative (downward S wave) in lead V_1, and positive (upright R′ wave) in leads V_5, V_6. Note that the *initial* part of the wide QRS complex (representing depolarization of the septum) is abnormal in LBBB (absent Q waves in V_5, V_6) (see reference text).

Importantly, the LBBB prolongs the QRS complex to greater than 0.12 second.

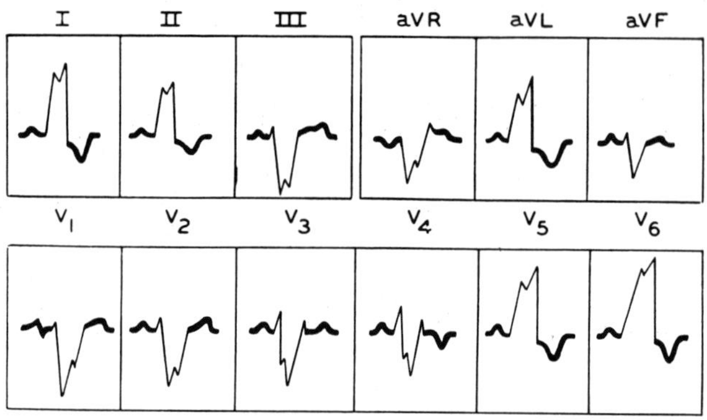

FIG 6–13.
Complete LBBB. Note the QRS duration greater than 0.12 second; deep S wave in V_1, V_2; RSR′ in V_5, V_6 with repolarization changes (also in leads I and aVL); and abnormal initial septal depolarization in V_5, V_6 (absent Q wave).

CRITERIA FOR COMPLETE LBBB

The ECG criteria for *complete LBBB* include the following:

1. QRS duration greater than 0.12 second.
2. RSR′ in the "left ventricular" leads V_5, V_6 (also I, aVL). The R′ represents late activation of the left ventricle as recorded in the "left ventricular" leads.
3. Wide or slurred S wave (negative deflection) in the "right ventricular" leads V_1, V_2. This represents late activation of the left ventricle as recorded in the "right ventricular" leads.
4. Ventricular repolarization changes (downsloping ST segment and inverted T wave—opposite direction to R′ wave) in leads V_5, V_6 (also I and aVL).
5. Late onset of intrinsicoid deflection (R peak time) in leads V_5, V_6 (greater than 0.06 second). This represents delayed onset of left ventricular activation.
6. Initial portion of QRS complex in leads V_5, V_6 (also I, aVL) is positive. No Q wave is present in these leads because of *abnormal septal depolarization* (see reference text).

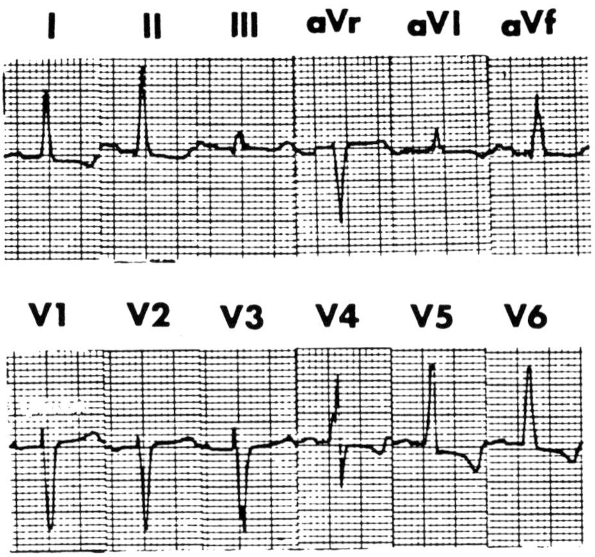

FIG 6–14.
Incomplete LBBB. Note the QRS duration between 0.10 and 0.12 second and the similar criteria for LBBB. This may also represent left ventricular hypertrophy.

INCOMPLETE LBBB

The ECG criteria for *incomplete LBBB* include the following:

1. QRS duration between 0.10 and 0.12 second.
2. RSR′ in leads V_5, V_6, (also I, aVL).
3. Broad S wave in leads V_1, V_2.
4. Late onset of intrinsicoid deflection (R peak time) in leads V_5, V_6 (greater than 0.06 second).

Note that incomplete LBBB resembles left ventricular hypertrophy (LVH) (see Chapter 8), and it may be difficult to differentiate between the two. In fact, both are often present at the same time.

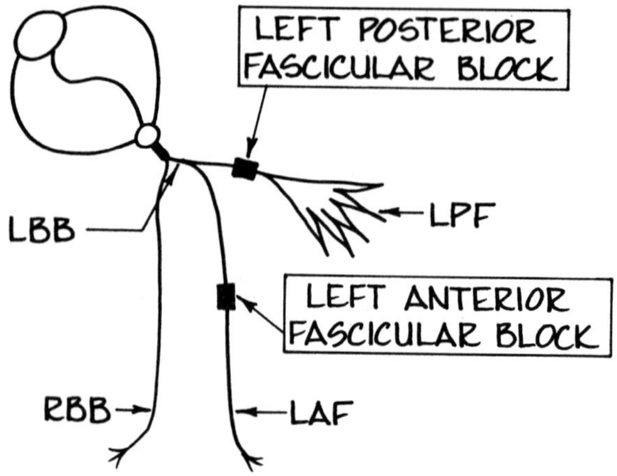

FIG 6–15.
Left posterior fascicular block and left anterior fascicular blocks. *LBB,* left bundle branch; *RBB,* right bundle branch; *LPF,* left posterior fascicle; *LAF,* left anterior fascicle.

FASCICULAR BLOCKS

The LBB divides relatively early into two major divisions termed anterior and posterior fascicles. The *left anterior fascicle* is long and thin and supplies the anterior and superior portions of the left ventricle. The *left posterior fascicle* is short and wide and supplies the posterior and inferior portions of the left ventricle through a fan-like array of conducting fibers.

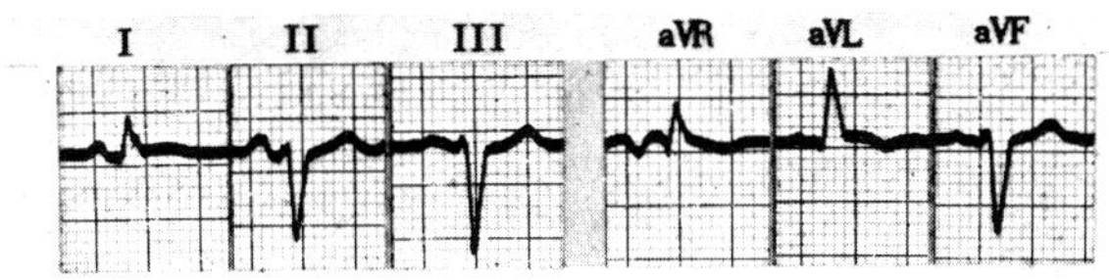

FIG 6–16.
Left anterior fascicular block. Note the marked left axis deviation (−45°); the small q and large R in *I, aVL,* and the small r and deep S in *II, III, aVF.*

LEFT ANTERIOR FASCICULAR BLOCK

The occurrence of LAFB indicates an interruption in activation of the anterior fascicle of the left bundle so that conduction proceeds initially through the posterior fascicle. The anterior and superior portions of the left ventricle are activated last. The ECG criteria for LAFB are derived primarily from the limb leads and include the following:

1. QRS duration between 0.08 and 0.11 second.
2. Left axis deviation (LAD) between −45° and −90°.
3. Small q wave and large R wave in leads I and aVL. The large R wave represents unopposed, late activation of the anterior and superior portions of the left ventricle.
4. Small r wave and deep S wave in leads II, III, and aVF.
5. Absence of other causes of LAD such as inferior myocardial infarction, hypertrophic subaortic stenosis, COPD, and Wolff-Parkinson-White syndrome (WPW) type B (see p. 136).

Additional findings of LAFB may include delayed onset of the intrinsicoid deflection (greater than 0.04 second) in leads I and aVL; repolarization changes in I and aVL; and small q wave with tall R wave in aVR.

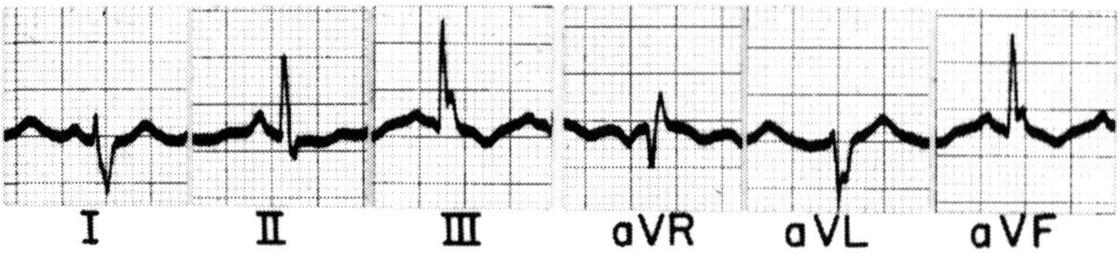

FIG 6–17.
Left posterior fascicular block. Note the marked right axis deviation (+120°); the small r and deep s in *I, aVL;* the small q and large R in *II, III, aVF;* and the prolonged QRS duration (0.11 second).

LEFT POSTERIOR FASCICULAR BLOCK

The occurrence of LPFB indicates an interruption in activation of the posterior fascicle of the left bundle. Conduction proceeds first through the anterior fascicle, leaving the posterior and inferior portions of the left ventricle to be activated last. Because the left posterior fascicle has a wide distribution of fibers and a double blood supply, LPFB is relatively uncommon.

The ECG criteria for LPFB are derived primarily from the limb leads and include the following:

1. QRS duration between 0.08 and 0.11 second.
2. Right axis deviation (RAD) between +90° and +180°.
3. Small q wave and large R wave in leads II, III, and aVF.
4. Small r wave and deep S wave in leads I and aVL.
5. Absence of other causes of RAD such as right ventricular hypertrophy (RVH), obstructive pulmonary disease, and lateral myocardial infarction.

Additional findings of LPFB may include delayed onset of intrinsicoid deflection (greater than 0.04 second) in leads II, III, and aVF, and repolarization changes in leads II, III, and aVF.

PEARLS

1. Episodes of sinus impulse dysfunction such as SA block, SA pause, or marked sinus bradycardia that alternate with episodes of supraventricular tachycardia are manifestations of sick sinus syndrome (see p. 143).

2. Mobitz type I (Wenckebach) AV block with a narrow QRS complex is relatively benign compared with Mobitz type II AV block with a wide QRS complex.

3. Acute myocardial infarction is difficult to diagnose in the presence of LBBB.

4. Be careful not to diagnose an old anterior myocardial infarction in the presence of LBBB, LVH, WPW syndrome, and pulmonary embolism. A Q wave or small R wave in leads V_1, V_2 is commonly present in these conditions and may resemble an old anterior myocardial infarction.

5. The normal initial septal depolarization vector (left to right) is unchanged in RBBB. In LBBB, the initial septal depolarization vector is reversed (right to left); the normal septal Q wave is absent in leads 1, aVL, V_5, V_6, and the Q wave of myocardial infarction may also be masked.

7 / Myocardial Ischemia, Injury, Infarction

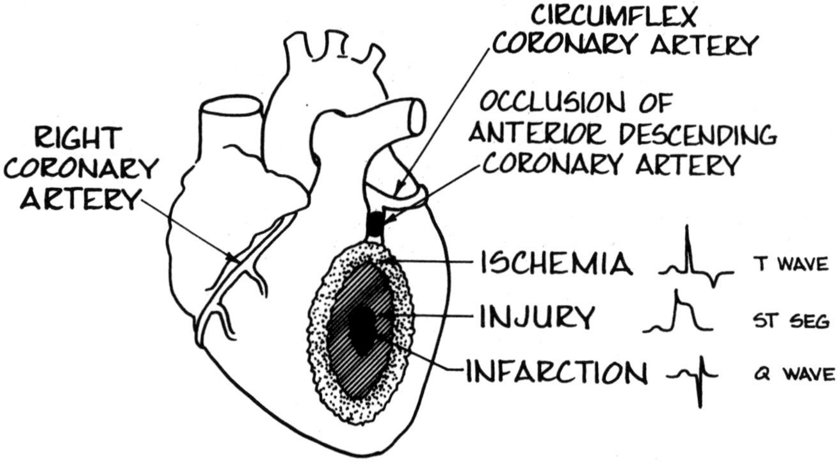

FIG 7–1.
Occlusion of the *anterior descending coronary artery* diagrammatically illustrating the three myocardial and ECG changes of acute *ischemia, injury,* and *infarction.*

When the coronary blood supply to the heart muscle is acutely compromised, three ECG changes may be recorded:

1. Ischemia (T wave change)
2. Injury (ST segment change)
3. Infarction (QRS change)

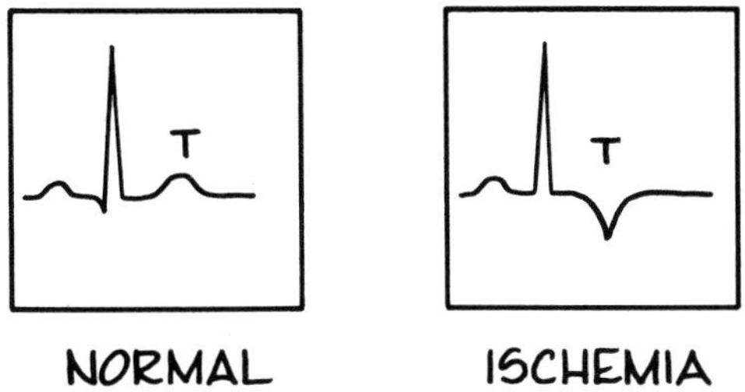

FIG 7–2.
Acute myocardial ischemia depicted by a symmetrically inverted T wave.

MYOCARDIAL ISCHEMIA

Myocardial ischemia is manifested by T wave changes in the ECG and denotes a temporary reduction of the blood supply to the myocardium. When the blood supply is restored, ischemia resolves and the T waves return to normal. If the blood supply is not restored, myocardial injury (ST segment change) or myocardial infarction (QRS change) may occur.

Acute myocardial ischemia is depicted by *symmetrical* inversion of the T wave (see figure). The normally upright T wave becomes inverted in those leads representing the area of ischemia. Note that in ischemia, the T wave inversion is symmetrical (*primary* T wave change) as opposed to the asymmetric T wave inversion in digitalis effect ("Dig. effect") (see p. 120) and ventricular strain (see p. 128) (*secondary* T wave change). See reference text.

If a patient has *preexisting T wave inversion,* acute myocardial ischemia may be depicted by reversion to a normal-appearing, upright T wave. In this case, when acute ischemia causes the T wave to revert to an upright morphology, the T wave may be falsely called "normal." This situation is described as *pseudonormalization* of the T wave. Previous as well as serial ECG tracings are important in diagnosing acute myocardial ischemia. The clinical history is extremely important.

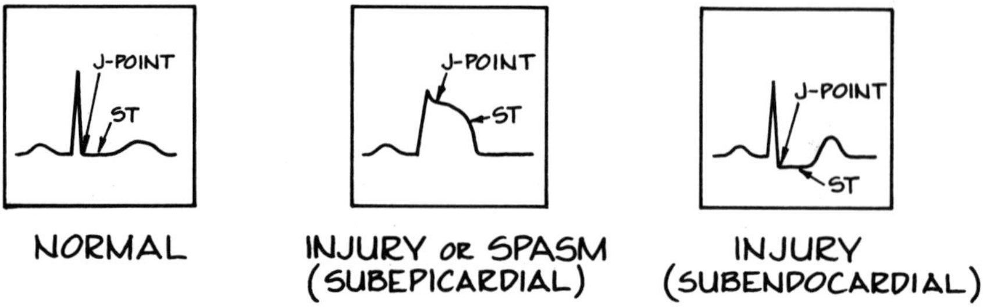

FIG 7–3.
Acute *subepicardial injury* (or *spasm*) depicted by elevated *J-point* and "coved" *ST* segment. Acute *subendocardial injury* is manifested by depressed *J-point* and *ST* segment.

MYOCARDIAL INJURY

Myocardial injury (ST segment change) denotes an acute reduction in the coronary blood supply causing injury to ventricular heart muscle. The injury may be reversible if the blood supply is promptly restored. If the blood supply is not reestablished within a short period of time, myocardial infarction (QRS change) may occur. In the ECG, acute myocardial injury is depicted by *elevation* or *depression* of the J point (beginning of the ST segment) and of the remaining ST segment.

Elevation of the ST segment occurs during *subepicardial* (outer ventricular wall) injury and represents reduction in blood supply of a major epicardial coronary artery. The ST elevation occurs in a convex direction upward, or "coved." Reciprocal changes ST depression) may occur in the leads representing the opposite side of the heart.

"Variant" or "Prinzmetal's" angina refers to angina caused by coronary artery spasm. This also causes a reduction in the blood supply of a major epicardial coronary artery and produces "coved" *ST elevation* in the affected areas. Coronary spasm is usually short-lived, and when it resolves, the ST segment returns to normal.

Depression of the ST segment occurs during *subendocardial* (inner ventricular wall) injury. During exercise testing, ST depression is an important indicator of coronary artery disease (see Fig 9–26, p. 147). If ST depression persists, it may result in subendocardial infarction (see Fig 7–7, p. 106).

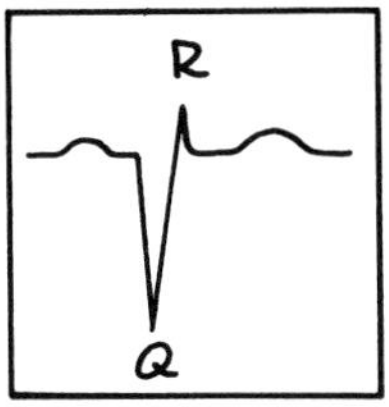

FIG 7–4.
Myocardial *infarction* depicted by a significant *Q* wave and loss of *R* wave height.

MYOCARDIAL INFARCTION

Myocardial infarction (QRS change) denotes death or necrosis of ventricular heart muscle when the compromised coronary blood supply is not reestablished. The heart muscle cells do not recover or regenerate; instead, a scar forms in the area of infarction.

Myocardial infarction is depicted by the appearance of Q waves. Note that *insignificant* Q waves are *normally* present in ECG leads I, aVL, V_5, and V_6 as a result of normal septal depolarization (see reference text). *Significiant* Q waves of myocardial infarction are Q waves that are greater than 0.04 second in duration and/or deeper than 25% of the height of the accompanying R wave.

The area of infarction is *electrically silent* and represents a "window" in the heart. The electrodes overlying the infarcted area "look through" the infarcted zone and record the depolarization forces moving in a direction away from the area of infarction. The Q wave, initial negative QRS deflection, represents the forces going away from the "dead" area of infarction.

In addition to Q waves, the loss of R wave height may also indicate infarction, because the height of the R wave is related to the amount of electrical activity of viable heart muscle. This is especially true for anterior myocardial infarction when "poor R wave progression" in the anterior chest leads (V_1, V_2, V_3, V_4) may indicate an old anterior infarction (see Fig 2–7,*C*).

LOCATION OF MYOCARDIAL INFARCTION

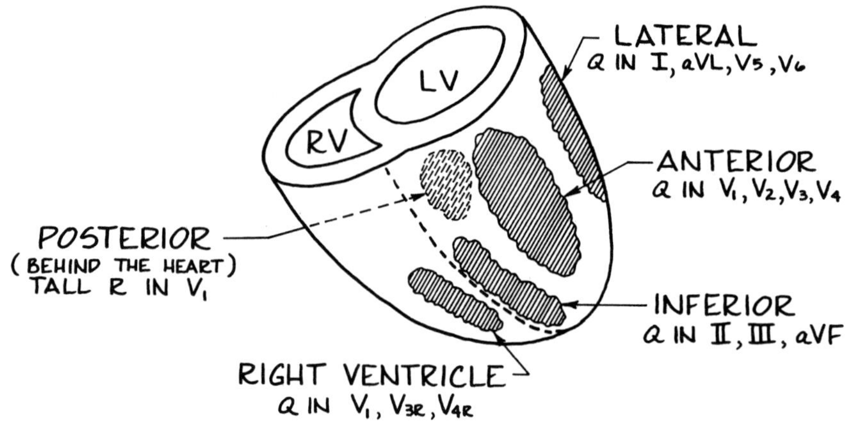

FIG 7–5.
Localization of the areas of infarction. *RV,* right ventricle; *LV,* left ventricle; V_{3R}, V_{4R}, right chest leads (see reference text).

LOCATION OF MYOCARDIAL INFARCTION

The Q waves of myocardial infarction appear in those ECG leads representing the areas of infarction. The locations and diagnostic ECG leads of myocardial infarction include the following:

1. *Anterior infarction:* Q waves in the anterior chest leads V_1, V_2, V_3, V_4.
2. *Inferior infarction:* Q waves in the inferior leads II, III, aVF.
3. *Lateral infarction:* Q waves in the lateral leads I, aVL, V_5, V_6.

Posterior infarction: tall R wave in lead V_1. Because the area of infarction is posterior, the depolarization waves in the anterior wall move unopposed and are recorded by the anterior V_1 electrode as an increased, tall R wave. A diagnostic criterion for posterior infarction is an R/S ratio in lead V_1 that is greater than one. Note also that *posterior infarction usually occurs in association with inferior and/or lateral myocardial infarction.*

5. *Right ventricular infarction:* Q wave or ST segment elevation in lead V_1 or right chest leads V_{3R}, V_{4R} (see reference text). *Right ventricular infarction usually occurs in association with inferior infarction.*

During acute myocardial infarction, injury (ST elevation) and ischemia (T wave changes) occur in the same areas of the heart and are seen in the same diagnostic ECG leads described for the Q waves.

EVOLUTION OF ACUTE MYOCARDIAL INFARCTION

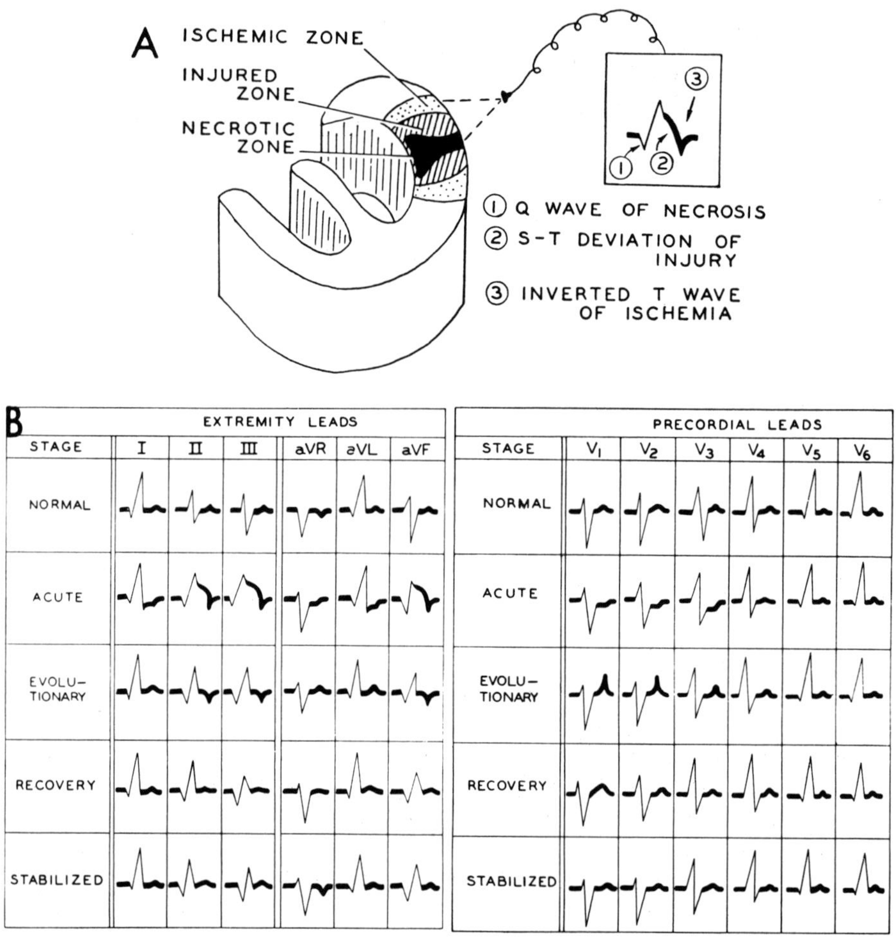

FIG 7–6.
A, the combined electrical patterns of acute *ischemia, injury,* and infarction recorded by a surface electrode. **B,** evolving changes of an acute inferior myocardial infarction. Note the ST, T, and Q wave changes during the acute stage in the inferior leads *(II, III, aVF).* Also note the reciprocal ST depression in the lateral and anterior leads *(I, aVL,* V_1, V_2, V_3*)* during the *acute* stage.

EVOLUTION OF ACUTE MYOCARDIAL INFARCTION

When a coronary artery becomes acutely obstructed, a progression of stages from ischemia to injury to infarction may be recorded in the ECG. Depending on the location, extent, and duration of the acute infarction, the involved leads may show T wave inversion (ischemia), ST elevation (injury), or Q waves (infarction). These are the classic ECG changes of an "evolving" myocardial infarction. The time period for each ECG change may be highly variable, and 1, 2, 3, or none of these ECG changes may be noted during an acute infarction (Fig 7–6,*A*). Serial tracings and the clinical history are important when evaluating an "evolving" myocardial infarction.

During acute infarction, the ST elevation may be associated with *reciprocal* ST depression in the ECG leads opposite to the area of infarction. For example (Fig 7–6,*B*), during acute inferior myocardial infarction, ST elevation in leads II, III, aVF is associated with reciprocal ST depression in the chest leads (V_1, V_2, V_3) and lateral leads (I, aVL).

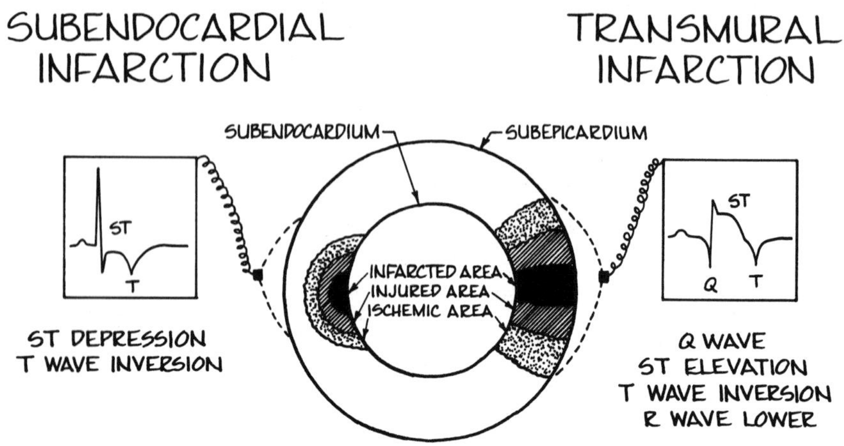

FIG 7–7.
Subendocardial (non Q wave) *infarction* diagrammatically depicted by *ST depression* and *T wave inversion* without a *Q wave. Transmural* (Q wave) infarction diagrammatically depicted by *ST elevation, T wave inversion,* and *Q wave.*

TRANSMURAL VS. SUBENDOCARDIAL INFARCTION

Transmural myocardial infarction (so-called "Q wave infarction") denotes death of myocardial tissue extending from the outer (subepicardial) portion of the ventricular wall to the inner (subendocardial) portion of the ventricular wall. This results from obstruction of one of the epicardial coronary arteries supplying an entire section of the wall of the affected ventricle. *Transmural infarction is depicted by Q waves in those ECG leads representing the area of infarction.*

The *subendocardial* (inner) layer of the ventricle is supplied by smaller branches of the major coronary arteries. Because the subendocardium is further from the major coronary arteries and because it is subjected to increased pressure during systole, it is more susceptible to the effects of the reduction in blood supply. In fact, the subendocardium may be the only area of myocardium that is affected by a reduction in blood flow resulting in subendocardial infarction.

Subendocardial infarction is a difficult ECG diagnosis to make. A Q wave does not occur. Instead, an initial pattern of ischemia (T wave change) with or without persistent ST depression is seen. The typical injury (ST elevation) and morphologic indications of infarction (Q wave) are absent. Subendocardial infarction is also termed *non-Q wave* infarction. In order to diagnose subendocardial infarction, serial tracings and knowledge of the entire clinical picture, including laboratory data, are very important.

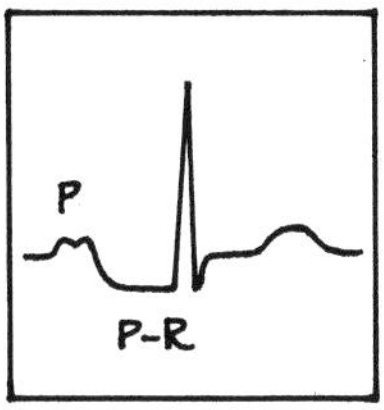

ATRIAL INFARCTION

FIG 7–8.
Atrial infarction depicted by change in *P* wave morphology and *P-R* segment depression.

ATRIAL INFARCTION

Infarction of the atria is not recognized commonly, but when found, it usually occurs in conjunction with inferior myocardial infarction. The diagnosis of atrial infarction is supported by one or more of the following criteria:

1. Change in P wave morphology
2. Elevation or depression of the P-R segment
3. Atrial arrhythmias (atrial fibrillation, atrial flutter, APCs)
4. Atrial conduction disturbances (SA block, AV block)

Because the atria are thin-walled chambers acting primarily as conduits, atrial infarction is usually not associated with the same hemodynamic consequences as ventricular infarction. In a compromised heart, however, the loss of the "atrial kick" (atrial contraction) may be significant.

8 / Atrial and Ventricular Hypertrophy

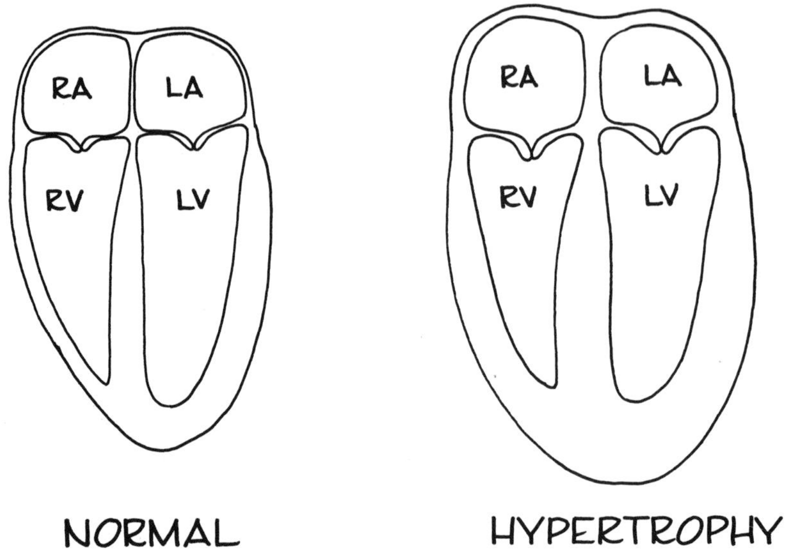

FIG 8–1.
Myocardial hypertrophy diagrammatically illustrated. Note the increase in thickness of the walls of both atria and ventricles. However, hypertrophy may be localized to a single chamber or combination of chambers. *RA,* right atrium; *LA,* left atrium; *RV,* right ventricle; *LV,* left ventricle.

Myocardial hypertrophy denotes increase in the thickness of the walls of the atria or ventricles. Hypertrophy should be differentiated from dilatation, which denotes increase in the internal diameter of the atria or ventricles. However, because the ECG manifestations of both conditions may be similar, they will be described under one heading of hypertrophy. The ECG interpretation of atrial or ventricular hypertrophy requires review of the anatomy and conducting system of the heart (see chapter 1).

The right atrium lies anterior to the left atrium. Atrial activation begins in the SA node, which is located in the superior and posterior part of the right atrium. Atrial depolarization proceeds first through the right atrium, then through the left atrium. Thus, right atrial activation is responsible for the initial part of the P wave, and left atrial activation is responsible for the terminal portion of the P wave. Depolarization of both atria is represented in the ECG by the P wave. The normal P wave is less than 0.11 second in duration and less than 2.5 mm in height.

The right ventricle lies anterior to the left ventricle. Because the left ventricle possesses three-to-four times the mass of the right ventricle, depolarization of the left ventricle produces the majority of the QRS deflection. Depolarization of both ventricles is represented in the ECG by the QRS complex, which is normally less than 0.10 second in duration.

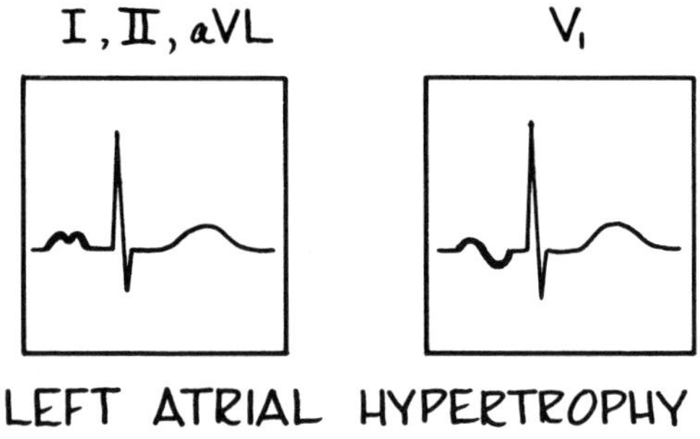

FIG 8–2.
Left atrial hypertrophy. Note the broad, notched P wave in *I, II, aVL* and the large terminal negative P wave deflection in V_1.

LEFT ATRIAL HYPERTROPHY

The ECG criteria for left atrial hypertrophy include the following:

1. Broad, notched, P wave greater than 0.11 second in duration in leads I, II, and aVL.
2. Large terminal negative P wave deflection (greater than 0.04 second) in chest lead V_1 representing the depolarization forces traveling posteriorly in the larger left atrium.
3. Leftward P wave axis (P wave axis between +30° and −30°).

Left atrial hypertrophy is also referred to as "P mitrale" because of the mitral valve diseases (mitral stenosis, mitral regurgitation) that are associated with this condition.

RIGHT ATRIAL HYPERTROPHY

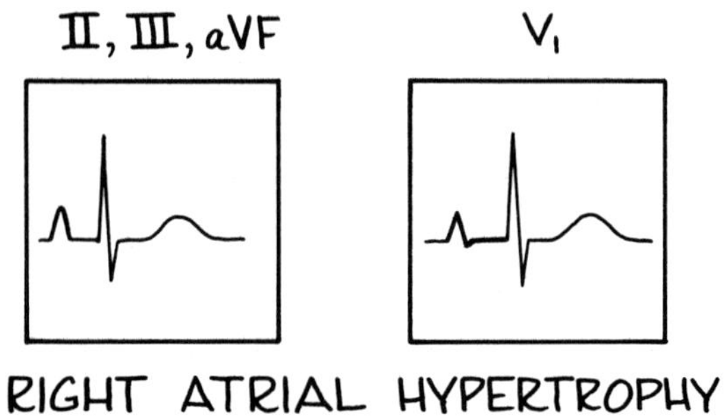

FIG 8–3.
Right atrial hypertrophy. Note the tall, peaked P wave in *II, III, aVF* and the large initial positive P wave deflection in V_1.

RIGHT ATRIAL HYPERTROPHY

The ECG criteria for right atrial hypertrophy include the following:

1. Tall, peaked P wave greater than 2.5 mm in height in leads II, III, aVF and large initial positive deflection of the P wave in lead V_1.
2. Rightward P wave axis (P wave axis between +75° and +90°).
3. Duration of P wave usually normal (less than 0.11 second).

Right atrial hypertrophy is also referred to as "P pulmonale" or "P congenitale" because of the pulmonary or congenital heart conditions, respectively, that are associated with this entity.

LEFT VENTRICULAR HYPERTROPHY (LVH)

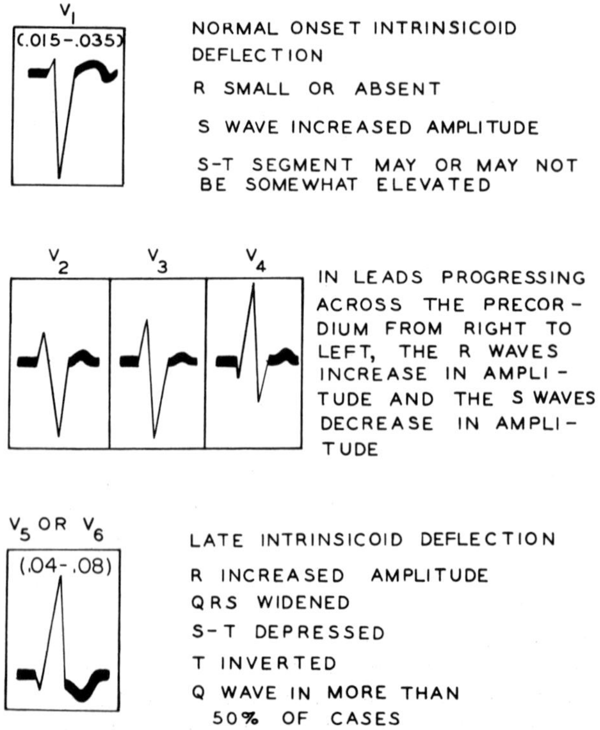

FIG 8–4.
Left ventricular hypertrophy (LVH) in the chest leads.

LEFT VENTRICULAR HYPERTROPHY (LVH)

The ECG criteria for LVH include the following:

1. Increased voltage of QRS complexes (most important criterion):
   a. R wave in V_5 or V_6 plus S wave in V_1 greater than 35 mm, or
   b. R wave in V_5 or V_6 greater than 26 mm, or
   c. R wave in aVL greater than 11 mm, or
   d. R wave in I plus S wave in III greater than 25 mm.

2. Repolarization changes (depressed ST segment and inverted T wave—opposite in direction to the R wave) in leads V_5, V_6 (and I, aVL).

3. Increased duration of QRS complexes. Because of the increased muscle mass, depolarization of the ventricles takes longer than normal and prolongs the QRS complex to between 0.10 and 0.12 second.

4. Left axis deviation (LAD) (QRS axis between −30° and −90°). This is secondary to the larger contribution of the increased left ventricular muscle mass.

5. Delayed onset of intrinsicoid deflection, R peak time, to greater than 0.06 second in left ventricular chest leads V_5, V_6 (see Fig 3–10). The onset of the intrinsicoid deflection, measured from the beginning of the QRS complex to the peak of the R wave, represents the time for the impulse to travel through the ventricles to the area that underlies the recording electrode. The increased left ventricular muscle mass prolongs this time interval.

3 POINTS ~ VOLTAGE

3 POINTS ~ ST SEGMENT, T WAVE CHANGES

(EXCEPTION: 1 POINT IF PATIENT IS TAKING DIGITALIS)

3 POINTS ~ LEFT ATRIAL HYPERTROPHY

2 POINTS ~ LEFT AXIS DEVIATION

1 POINT ~ WIDENED QRS

1 POINT ~ DELAYED INTRINSICOID DEFLECTION

FIG 8–5.
Estes criteria for left ventricular hypertrophy (LVH). Five or more points is *diagnostic of LVH;* four points is *probable LVH.*

ESTES CRITERIA FOR LVH

A point scoring system developed by Estes is useful for diagnosing LVH:

1. Three points (voltage):
   a. R wave or S wave in any limb lead of 20 mm or more, or
   b. S wave in V_1, V_2, V_3, of 25 mm or more, or
   c. R wave in V_4, V_5, V_6 of 25 mm or more.
2. Three points (repolarization changes): ST depression and T wave inversion opposite in direction to the QRS deflection in leads V_5, V_6.

Note: Only one point is given if the patient is taking digoxin and has these repolarization changes.

3. Three points: large terminal negative P wave deflection greater than 0.04 second in chest lead V_1 representing associated left atrial hypertrophy.
4. Two points: left axis deviation greater than $-15°$.
5. One point: increased QRS duration equal to or greater than 0.09 second.
6. One point: delayed onset of the intrinsicoid deflection to greater than 0.04 second in the left chest leads (V_5, V_6).

The maximum number of points is 13. Five or more points is diagnostic of LVH. Four points indicates probable LVH. As can be seen from above, the most important criteria are increased QRS voltage, repolarization changes, and left atrial hypertrophy.

RIGHT VENTRICULAR HYPERTROPHY (RVH)

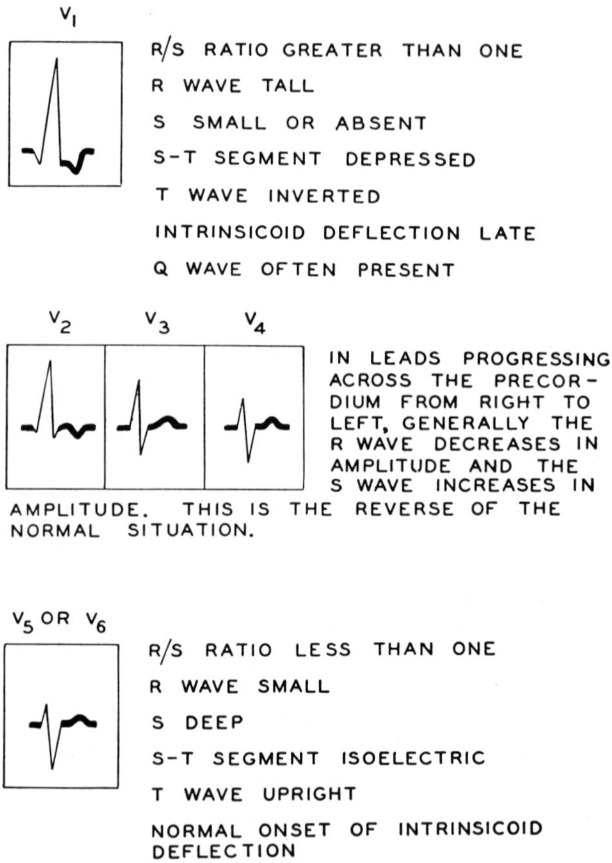

FIG 8–6.
Right ventricular hypertrophy (RVH) in the chest leads.

RIGHT VENTRICULAR HYPERTROPHY (RVH)

The diagnosis of RVH can be difficult. The ECG criteria for RVH include the following:

1. Right axis deviation (RAD) (axis between +90° and +180°). This is secondary to the increased right ventricular muscle mass and shift of the heart position. RAD is an important criterion for diagnosing RVH.
2. Increased voltage of QRS complexes:
   a. R/S ratio in V_1 is greater than one, or
   b. R wave in V_1 plus S wave in V_5 or V_6 is equal to or greater than 10.5 mm, or
   c. R wave in V_1 is greater than 7 mm, or
   d. R wave in aVR is greater than 5 mm, or
   e. S wave in V_1 is less than 2 mm, or
   f. prominent S wave in V_5, V_6.
3. Repolarization changes (depressed ST segment and inverted T wave—opposite in direction to the R wave) in right chest leads V_1, V_2.
4. Mild increase in duration of QRS complexes. This represents prolonged depolarization because of RVH. The QRS duration may measure 0.10 second or more.
5. Delayed onset of intrinsicoid deflection to greater than 0.04 second in right precordial leads V_1, V_2.
6. Incomplete RBBB pattern (rSR′ in V_1).
7. Small Q wave in chest lead V_1.

PEARLS

1. Q waves in leads V_1, V_2, V_3 may be seen in LVH and may be mistaken for an old anterior myocardial infarction.

2. RVH may be masked by complete RBBB. (See reference text.).

3. In RVH, the chest leads show reversal of usual QRS chest pattern with tall R in right chest leads (V_1, V_2) and deep S in left chest leads (V_5, V_6), or simply rS complexes in all the chest leads.

9 / Drugs, Electrolytes, Miscellaneous

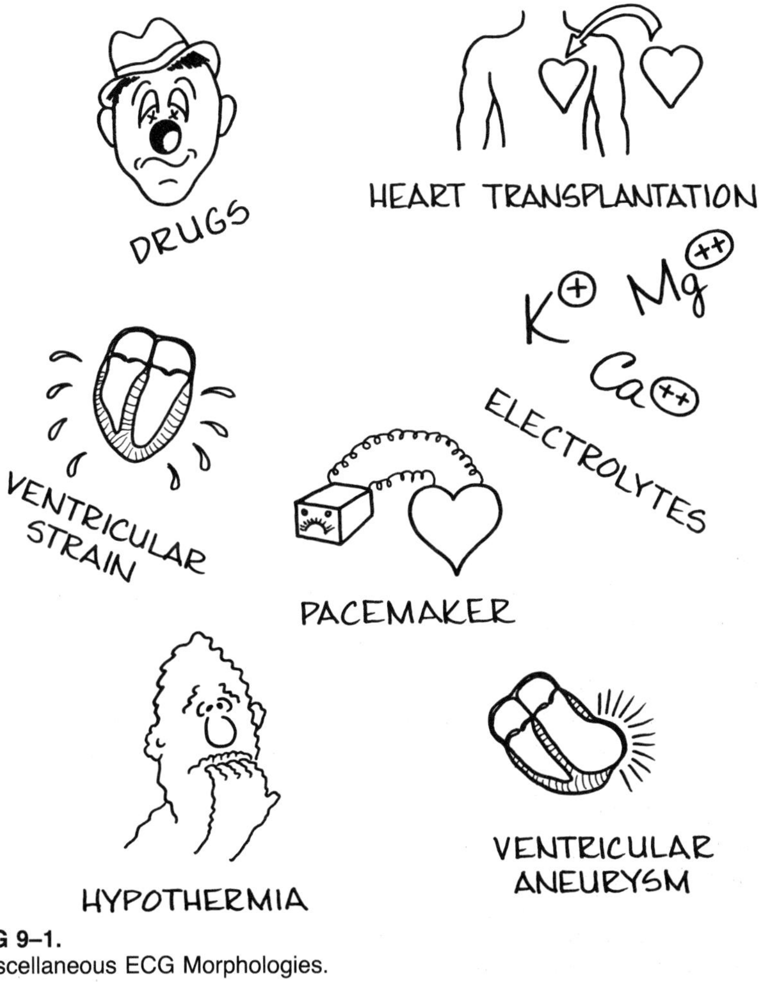

FIG 9–1.
Miscellaneous ECG Morphologies.

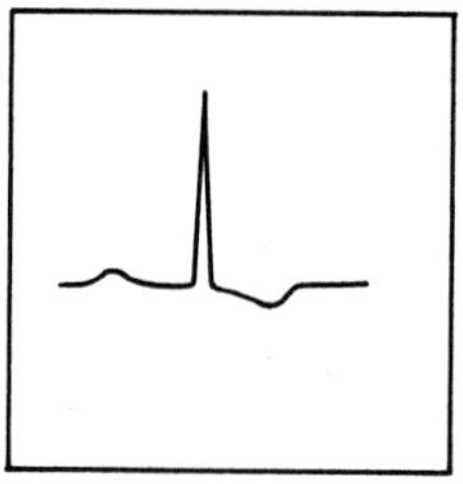

FIG 9–2.
"Dig. effect." ECG manifestations include *ST depression, T wave inversion, shortening* of the *Q-T interval,* and mild lengthening of the *P-R interval.*

DIGITALIS EFFECT ("DIG. EFFECT")

Digoxin is a commonly prescribed cardiac drug. Like other digitalis preparations, it frequently causes ECG changes primarily in the repolarization phase (ST segment, T wave), which are termed "Dig. effect." The ECG changes seen with "Dig. effect" include the following:

1. Depressed ST segments in leads where the main QRS deflections are upright and elevated ST segments where the main QRS deflections are downward. The depressed ST segments appear to "sag" as in ventricular hypertrophy and "strain."
2. Flattened or inverted T waves. These changes are similar to and can mask changes of ischemia or hypertrophy.
3. Shortening of the Q-T interval.
4. Modest lengthening of the P-R interval.

The ECG changes of "Dig. effect" are frequent findings in patients who are taking digoxin and *are not indicative of toxicity.* "Dig. toxic" arrhythmias are discussed on following page.

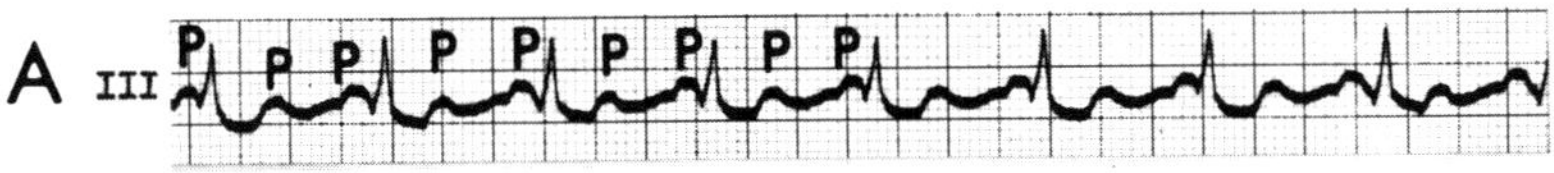

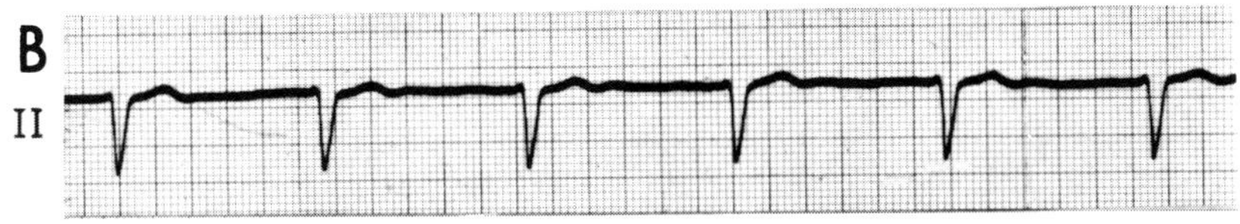

FIG 9–3.
A, atrial tachycardia with block secondary to "Dig. toxicity." Note the regularity of the *P* waves (rate 180) with 2:1 AV conduction, ventricular rate of 90. Every other P wave is buried in the T wave. **B,** junctional rhythm at a regular rate of 52 with underlying atrial fibrillation during treatment with digoxin. This is a type of AV dissociation, and it is indicative of "Dig. toxicity." Note the slight undulation of the baseline characteristic of atrial fibrillation.

DIGITALIS TOXICITY ("DIG. TOXICITY")

Digoxin in excess can cause toxic effects including serious arrhythmias. Early symptoms of "Dig. toxicity" include nausea, vomiting, and anorexia. Arrhythmias of "Dig. toxicity" include the following:

1. Atrial arrhythmias: sinus bradycardia, SA block, APCs, *atrial tachycardia with AV block* (traditionally a common "Dig. toxic" arrhythmia, Fig 9–3,*A*).
2. AV junctional arrhythmias: first-degree AV block (prolonged P-R interval), second-degree AV block (commonly Mobitz type I or Wenckebach), third-degree AV block, JPCs, junctional rhythm (rate 40–60), accelerated junctional rhythm (rate 60–150).
3. Ventricular arrhythmias: VPCs, bigeminy, ventricular tachycardia that may be bidirectional, ventricular flutter, ventricular fibrillation.

Note that during treatment of atrial fibrillation with digoxin, regularization of rhythm *(junctional rhythm)* should alert one to the possibility of "Dig. toxicity" (Fig 9–3,*B*).

Treatment of "Dig. toxicity" includes discontinuation of digoxin, potassium supplementation, and pacemaker if hemodynamically necessary.

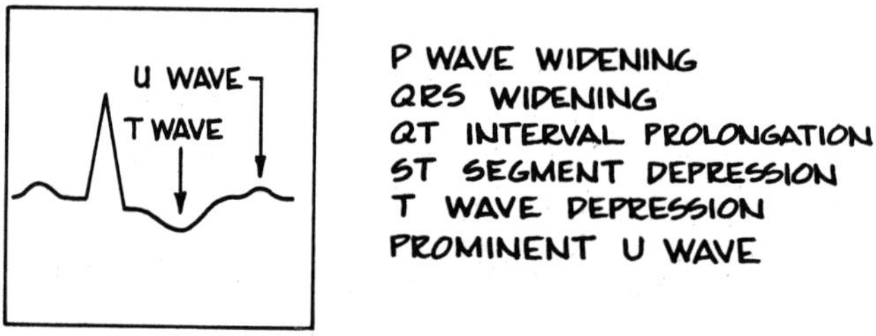

FIG 9–4.
ECG effects of type I antiarrhythmic drug therapy.

QUINIDINE, PROCAINAMIDE, DISOPYRAMIDE EFFECTS

Type I antiarrhythmic drugs such as quinidine, procainamide, and disopyramide may produce ECG changes that include the following:

1. Increase in duration of the Q-T interval (very important).
2. Widening of the P wave and QRS complex.
3. Repolarization changes of ST depression and T wave inversion in the left ventricular leads (I, aVL, V_4, V_5, V_6).
4. Prominent U wave.

Toxicity from these antiarrhythmic drugs may occur when the QRS complex or Q-T interval widens by greater than 25% compared with the baseline QRS and Q-T values. These antiarrhythmic drugs may at times cause toxic arrhythmias that include the following:

1. Atrial arrhythmias: SA block, intra-atrial block (widening of the P wave).
2. AV block: first-degree, second-degree, and third-degree block.
3. Ventricular arrhythmias: VPCs, idioventricular rhythm, ventricular tachycardia, ventricular fibrillation.
4. Torsade de pointes: associated with prolongation of the Q-T interval (see p. 71). Torsade de pointes is usually short-lived and terminates spontaneously, or it may deteriorate into ventricular fibrillation. Note that "quinidine syncope" is believed to be caused by the ventricular arrhythmias of torsade de pointes and/or ventricular fibrillation.

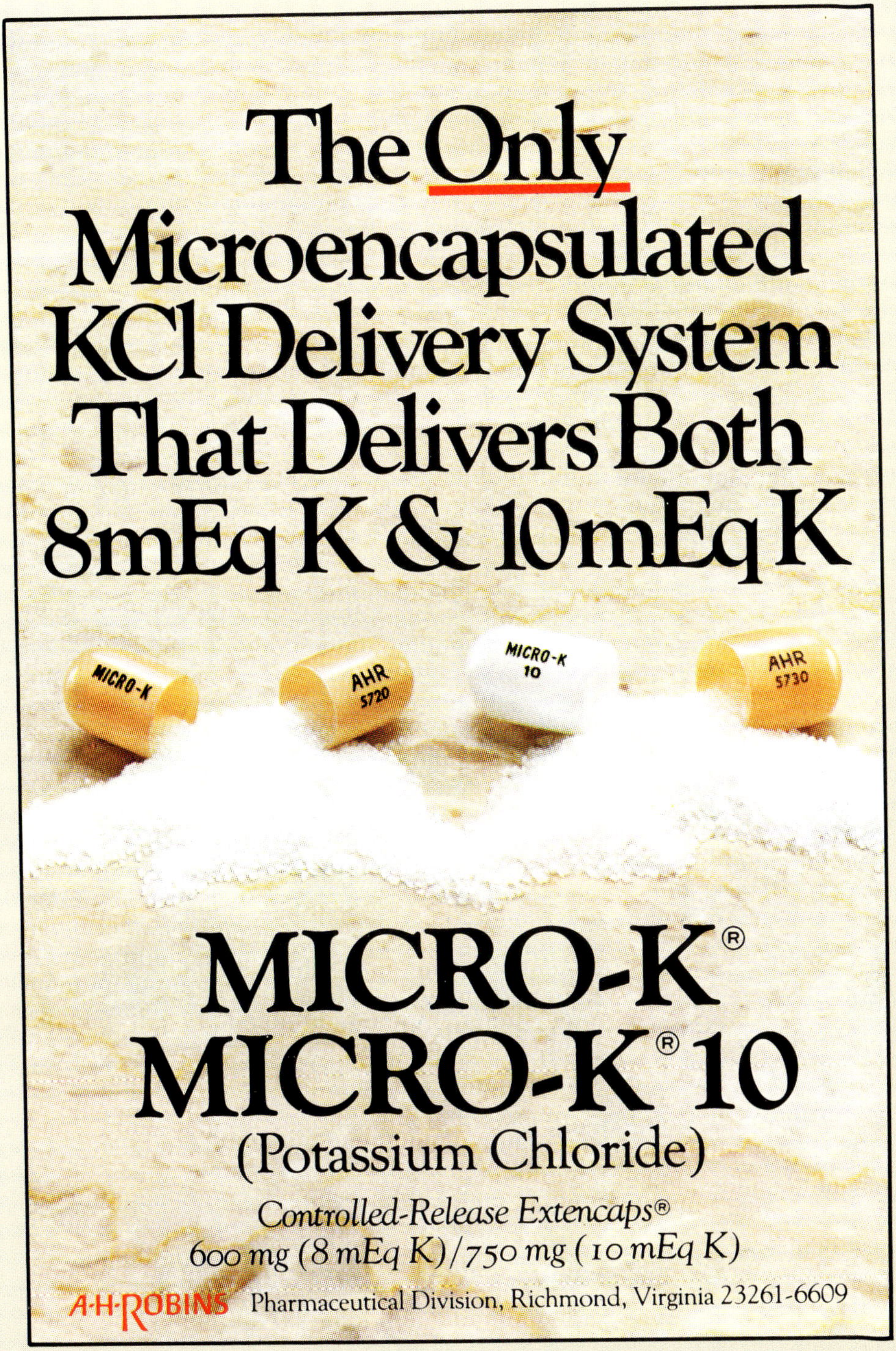

Please see prescribing information on the following page.

MICRO-K®

(Potassium Chloride)

The following is a brief summary only. Before prescribing, see complete prescribing information in Micro-K product labeling.

Indications: Because of reports of intestinal and gastric ulceration and bleeding with slow-release potassium chloride preparations, these drugs should be reserved for those patients who cannot tolerate or refuse to take liquid or effervescent potassium preparations or for patients in whom there is a problem of compliance with these preparations.

1. For therapeutic use in patients with hypokalemia with or without metabolic alkalosis; in digitalis intoxication and in patients with hypokalemic familial periodic paralysis.
2. For prevention of potassium depletion when the dietary intake of potassium is inadequate in the following conditions: patients receiving digitalis and diuretics for congestive heart failure; hepatic cirrhosis with ascites; states of aldosterone excess with normal renal function; potassium-losing nephropathy, and certain diarrheal states.
3. The use of potassium salts in patients receiving diuretics for uncomplicated essential hypertension is often unnecessary when such patients have a normal dietary pattern. Serum potassium should be checked periodically, however, and, if hypokalemia occurs, dietary supplementation with potassium-containing foods may be adequate to control milder cases. In more severe cases, supplementation with potassium salts may be indicated.

Contraindications: Potassium supplements are contraindicated in patients with hyperkalemia since a further increase in serum potassium concentration in such patients can produce cardiac arrest. Hyperkalemia may complicate any of the following conditions: chronic renal failure, systemic acidosis such as diabetic acidosis, acute dehydration, extensive tissue breakdown as in severe burns, adrenal insufficiency, or the administration of a potassium-sparing diuretic (e.g., spironolactone, triamterene).

Wax-matrix potassium chloride preparations have produced esophageal ulceration in certain cardiac patients with esophageal compression due to an enlarged left atrium.

All solid dosage forms of potassium supplements are contraindicated in any patient in whom there is cause for arrest or delay in tablet passage through the gastrointestinal tract. In these instances, potassium supplementation should be with a liquid preparation.

Warnings: *Hyperkalemia.* In patients with impaired mechanisms for excreting potassium, the administration of potassium salts can produce hyperkalemia and cardiac arrest. This occurs most commonly in patients given potassium by the intravenous route but may also occur in patients given potassium orally. Potentially fatal hyperkalemia can develop rapidly and be asymptomatic.

The use of potassium salts in patients with chronic renal disease, or any other condition which impairs potassium excretion, requires particularly careful monitoring of the serum potassium concentration and appropriate dosage adjustments.

Interaction with Potassium-Sparing Diuretics. Hypokalemia should not be treated by the concomitant administration of potassium salts and a potassium-sparing diuretic (e.g., spironolactone or triamterene), since the simultaneous administration of these agents can produce severe hyperkalemia.

Gastrointestinal lesions. Potassium chloride tablets have produced stenotic and/or ulcerative lesions of the small bowel and deaths, in addition to upper gastrointestinal bleeding. These lesions are caused by a high localized concentration of potassium ion in the region of a rapidly dissolving tablet which injures the bowel wall and thereby produces obstruction, hemorrhage, or perforation.

Micro-K Extencaps contain microcapsules which disperse upon dissolution of the hard gelatin capsule. The microcapsules are formulated to provide a controlled release of potassium chloride. The dispersibility of the microcapsules and the controlled release of ions from the microcapsules are intended to minimize the possibility of a high local concentration near the gastrointestinal mucosa and the ability of the KCl to cause stenosis or ulceration. Other means of accomplishing this (e.g., incorporation of KCl into a wax matrix) have reduced the frequency of such lesions to less than one per 100,000 patient years (compared to 40–50 per 100,000 patient years with enteric-coated KCl), but have not eliminated them. The frequency of GI lesions with Micro-K Extencaps is, at present, unknown. Micro-K Extencaps should be discontinued immediately and the possibility of bowel obstruction or perforation considered if severe vomiting, abdominal pain, distention, or gastrointestinal bleeding occurs.

Metabolic Acidosis. Hypokalemia in patients with metabolic *acidosis* should be treated with an alkalinizing potassium salt such as potassium bicarbonate, potassium citrate, or potassium acetate.

Precautions: The diagnosis of potassium depletion is ordinarily made by demonstrating hypokalemia in a patient with a clinical history suggesting some cause for potassium depletion. In interpreting the serum potassium level, the physician should bear in mind that acute alkalosis per se can produce hypokalemia in the absence of a deficit in total body potassium, while acute acidosis per se can increase the serum potassium concentration into the normal range even in the presence of a reduced total body potassium. The treatment of potassium depletion, particularly in the presence of cardiac disease, renal disease, or acidosis, requires careful attention to acid-base balance and appropriate monitoring of serum electrolytes, the electrocardiogram, and the clinical status of the patient.

Adverse Reactions: The most common adverse reactions to oral potassium salts are nausea, vomiting, abdominal discomfort, and diarrhea. These symptoms are due to irritation of the gastrointestinal tract and may be minimized by taking the dose with meals or by reducing the dose.

Intestinal bleeding, ulceration, perforation and obstruction have been reported in patients treated with solid dosage forms of potassium salts and may occur with Micro-K Extencaps (see Contraindications and Warnings).

One of the most severe adverse effects of potassium supplementation is hyperkalemia (see Contraindications, Warnings, and Overdosage).

Skin rash has been reported rarely with potassium preparations.

Rev. February 1985

A·H·ROBINS Pharmaceutical Division, Richmond, Virginia 23261-6609

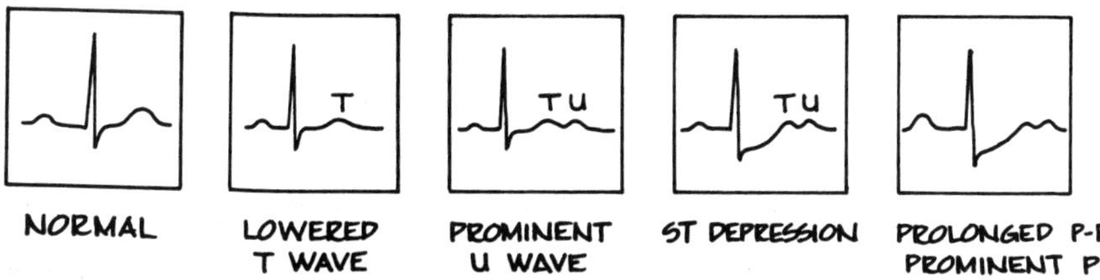

FIG 9–6.
ECG patterns of hypokalemia sequentially as potassium level decreases.

HYPOKALEMIA

Hypokalemia (low levels of serum potassium) causes the following ECG manifestations listed sequentially as potassium level decreases:

1. Lowering and inversion of T wave.
2. Prominent U wave.
3. ST depression.
4. Prominent P wave and prolongation of P-R interval.
5. Atrial and ventricular arrhythmias including ventricular tachycardia and ventricular fibrillation.

Treatment of hypokalemia is potassium administration and correction of the underlying cause.

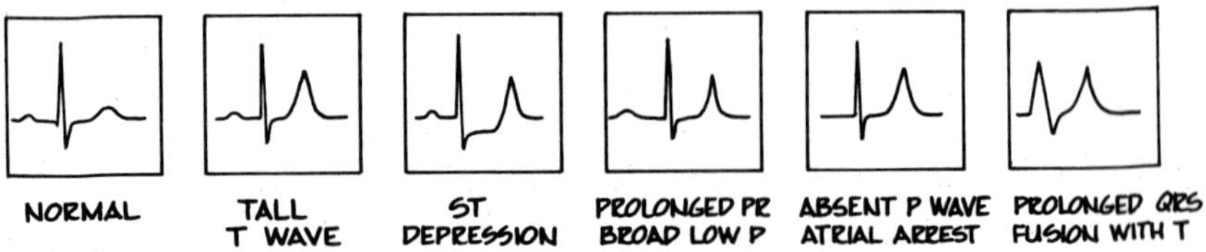

FIG 9–5.
ECG patterns of hyperkalemia sequentially as potassium level increases.

HYPERKALEMIA

Hyperkalemia (high levels of serum potassium) causes the following ECG manifestations listed sequentially as potassium level increases:

1. Tall, symmetrically peaked T wave.
2. ST depression.
3. P-R prolongation, widening and flattening of P wave.
4. P wave disappearance (atrial arrest).
5. QRS widening and fusion with tall T wave.
6. Ventricular tachycardia, ventricular flutter, ventricular fibrillation, ventricular standstill ("straight-line").

Treatment of hyperkalemia includes discontinuation of potassium, administration of calcium for toxic arrhythmias, glucose with insulin, bicarbonate, and sodium-potassium exchange resin (Kayexalate).

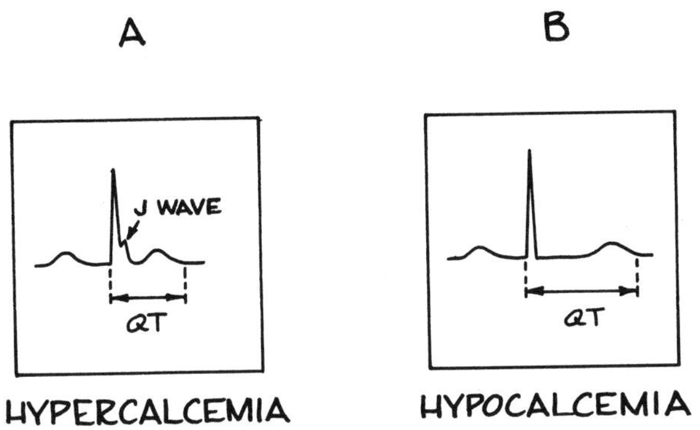

FIG 9–7.
A, ECG changes in *hypercalcemia,* shortening of the *QT* interval primarily by shortening of the ST segment. A *J wave* may also be seen. **B,** *hypocalcemia,* lengthening of the *QT* interval primarily by lengthening of the ST segment.

HYPERCALCEMIA, HYPOCALCEMIA

Hypercalcemia (high levels of serum calcium) causes shortening of the Q-T interval primarily by shortening the ST segment. There may also be prolongation of the P-R interval and QRS complex. The J wave, found in hypothermia (see following page), has also been reported in patients with hypercalcemia. Atrial or ventricular arrhythmias, especially in patients taking digoxin, may occur with hypercalcemia.

Hypocalcemia (low levels of serum calcium) causes lengthening of the Q-T interval primarily by lengthening the ST segment. It may cause atrial or ventricular arrhythmias including torsade de pointes (see p. 71).

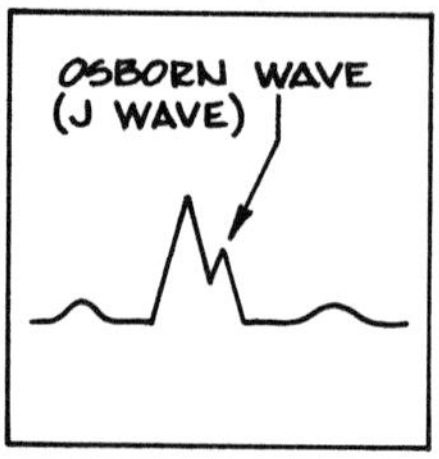

FIG 9–8.
ECG changes in Hypothermia. The *Osborn wave (J wave)* is frequently seen.

HYPOTHERMIA

Hypothermia (low body temperature) is occasionally observed in patients during freezing weather under adverse conditions. Hypothermia is also used in conjunction with cardiac operations. The ECG manifestations of hypothermia include the following:

1. Sinus bradycardia (35°–37° C).
2. Prolongation of P-R interval, QRS complex, ST segment, Q-T interval (30°–35° C).
3. *Osborn or O wave or J wave* (below 30° C). This wave or deflection appears at the end of ventricular depolarization (at the end of the QRS complex) and is characteristic of hypothermia.
4. Ventricular arrhythmias: VPCs, ventricular tachycardia, ventricular fibrillation (below 30° C).

Note that ventricular arrhythmias may occur during the rewarming process as well.

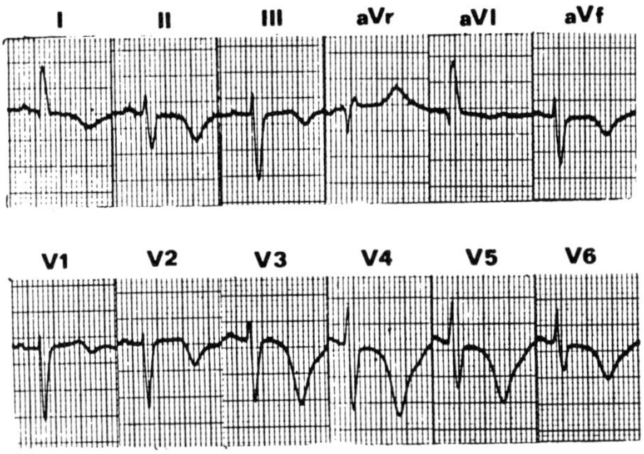

FIG 9–9.
ECG "CVA pattern." Observe the wide, deeply inverted T waves and prolonged Q-T interval in this patient with an intracerebral hemorrhage.

ECG CHANGES IN CEREBROVASCULAR ACCIDENTS (CVA)

Frequently, ECG changes occur in association with strokes, ruptured cerebral aneurysms, subarachnoid hemorrhages, and other central neurologic lesions. The ECG changes occur primarily during ventricular repolarization and are believed to be mediated through the autonomic nervous system and altered sympathetic tone. The ECG abnormalities include the following:

1. Abnormal and widened T waves that may be deeply inverted or tall and peaked.
2. Prominent U waves.
3. Prolonged Q-T interval.

These changes are termed "CVA pattern" and usually resolve with time.

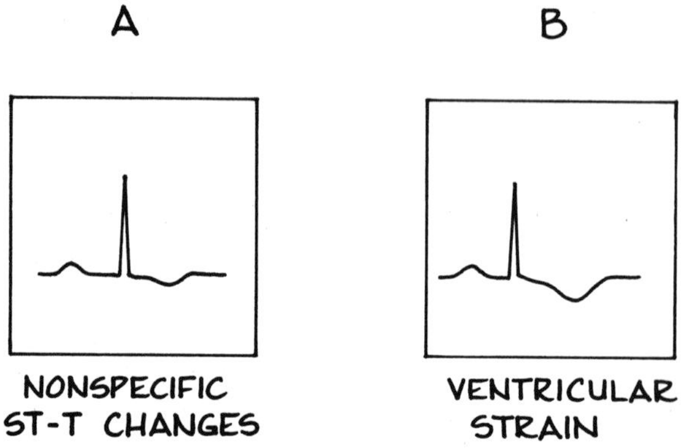

FIG 9–10.
A, ECG morphology of *nonspecific ST-T changes.* **B,** *ventricular strain.* In *ventricular strain,* the ST-T changes are similar to, but more pronounced than, *nonspecific ST-T changes.*

NONSPECIFIC ST-T CHANGES

Ventricular 'Strain'

Nonspecific or nondiagnostic ST-T changes is a commonly used ECG term for abnormal ventricular repolarization when a specific diagnosis cannot be made. The ECG displays mild downsloping and depression of the ST segment with lowering or inversion of the T wave (Fig 9–10,*A*).

Ventricular "strain" pattern is an exaggeration of the ECG findings of nonspecific ST-T changes. It is characterized by downsloping and depression of the ST segment with an asymmetrically inverted T wave (Fig 9–10,*B*). These ST and T changes usually appear in the left ventricular leads (I, aVL, V_4, V_5, V_6) without associated findings of increased QRS voltage, prolonged QRS duration, or clinical evidence of acute myocardial ischemia.

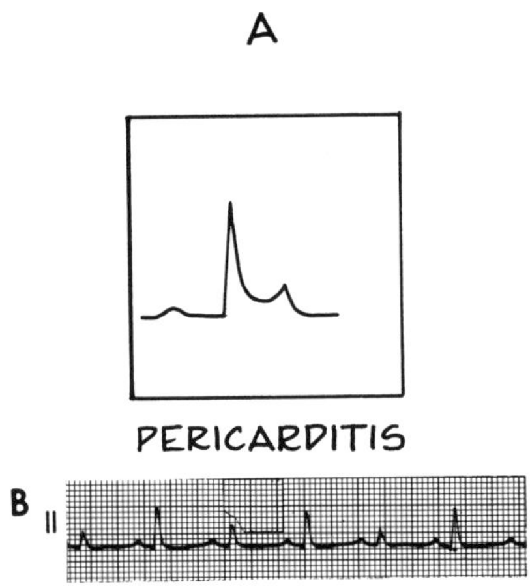

FIG 9–11.
A, ECG changes in pericarditis. The ST elevation is concave in an upward direction and is diffuse, not localized, in certain leads as in acute myocardial infarction. **B,** QRS electrical alternans. Note the alteration in QRS height in every other beat in this patient with a large pericardial effusion.

PERICARDITIS

Pericardial Effusion

Pericarditis denotes inflammation of the lining surrounding the heart. Acute pericarditis is manifested by ST elevation in most of the leads in the ECG (except lead aVR), representing the widespread nature of the cardiac involvement. The ST elevation is concave in an upward direction (Fig 9–11,*A*) and is due to injury to the subepicardial (outer) muscle layer of the heart next to the inflamed pericardium. The T wave remains upright during the acute phase.

As pericarditis resolves, the ST segments return to the baseline. The T waves subsequently become inverted. The T wave inversion may persist for weeks to months before returning to baseline.

The ST segment changes of acute pericarditis can be difficult to differentiate from acute myocardial infarction. However, in acute myocardial infarction, the ST elevation is usually *localized* to a few leads and is usually convex in an upward direction (see p. 100). Also, the T waves are inverted early in acute myocardial infarction. In addition to the ECG, the clinical history and physical examination are important in differentiating pericarditis from acute myocardial infarction.

Pericardial effusion (fluid surrounding the heart) may or may not be associated with pericarditis. The ECG manifestations of pericardial effusion include (1) decreased QRS voltage and (2) ventricular *electrical alternans* (alteration of the QRS height every other beat) (Fig 9–11,*B*).

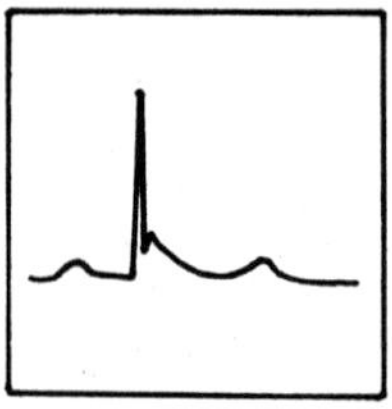

FIG 9–12.
ECG changes in early repolarization, a normal variant. In serial tracings, there are no changes in the elevated ST segments. Note the elevated J point with a small notch.

EARLY REPOLARIZATION

Early repolarization is characterized by ST elevation that is a *normal* ECG variant in young healthy individuals. It simulates and may be confused with the ST elevation of acute myocardial injury and acute pericarditis.

The ECG findings of early repolarization include the following:

1. Elevated J point with a small notch at the J point.
2. Elevated ST segment, concave upward.
3. Biphasic or inverted T wave (may or may not be present).
4. More commonly seen in young black males.

In diagnosing early repolarization, the clinical history is very important. Comparison with old ECGs and obtaining serial tracings may be necessary to show no change or evolution of the ST elevation.

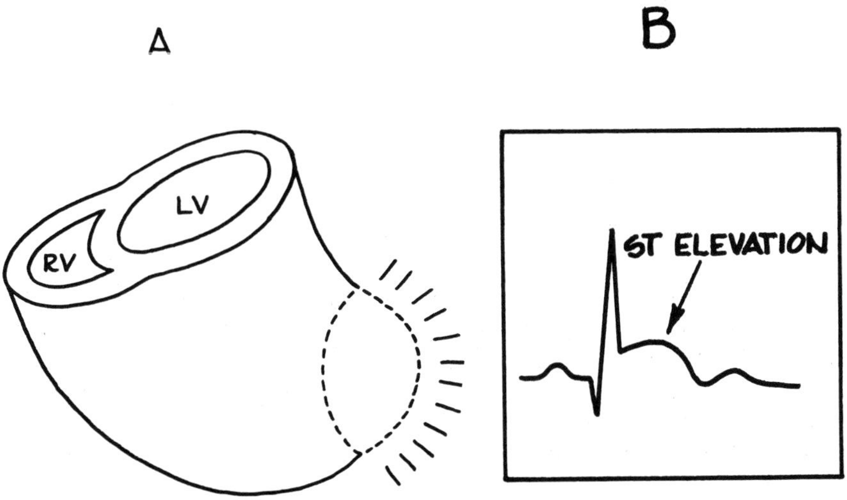

FIG 9–13.
A, ventricular aneurysm is an outpouching of scarred heart tissue. *RV,* right ventricle; *LV,* left ventricle. **B,** persistent convex *ST elevation* seen in ventricular aneurysm.

VENTRICULAR ANEURYSM

Ventricular aneurysm is an outpouching of the heart that occurs in the area of a previous myocardial infarction (Fig 9–13,*A*). It is comprised primarily of scar tissue. The ECG displays *persistent* abnormal ST elevation in those leads representing the area of the aneurysm. The ST elevation is convex upward and is identical to that of acute myocardial injury (Fig 9–13,*B*). However with ventricular aneurysm, the ST elevation persists for weeks, months, or years.

Metastatic tumors in the heart muscle may also produce persistently abnormal ST elevation.

PULMONARY EMBOLISM

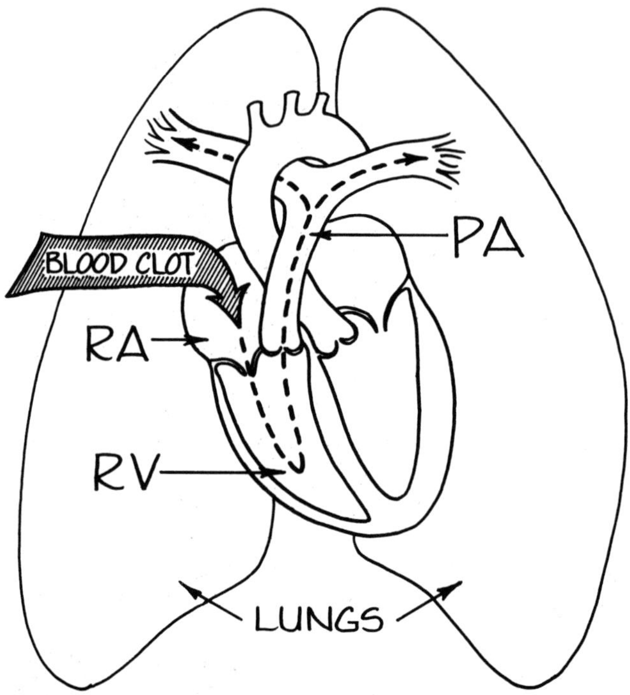

FIG 9–14.
Pulmonary embolism. A *blood clot* travels to the right atrium *(RA),* right ventricle *(RV),* pulmonary artery *(PA),* and into the *lungs.* The ECG manifestations of pulmonary embolism are due to the increase in pulmonary artery pressure and acute strain on the heart, especially on the right atrium and right ventricle. See next page for acute ECG changes.

PULMONARY EMBOLISM

Pulmonary embolism occurs when a blood clot becomes lodged in the circulation of the lungs. This causes the right atrium and right ventricle to work harder against a higher pressure in the lungs. The ECG may show one or more changes characteristic of pulmonary embolism, which include the following:

1. Sinus tachycardia and other transient supraventricular arrhythmias such as atrial fibrillation, atrial flutter, and PAT.
2. P pulmonale (tall P wave in leads II, III, aVF). This results from strain and dilatation of the right atrium.
3. RBBB (incomplete or complete). This results from strain and dilatation of the right ventricle.
4. ST depression and T wave inversion in the right precordial leads (V_1, V_2). This results from increased strain on the right ventricle.
5. RAD. This results from dilatation and strain of the right ventricle and shifting of the electrical position of the heart.
6. Sudden appearance of ST changes, T wave changes, and/or Q waves in the inferior and/or anterior leads simulating acute inferior and/or anterior myocardial infarction. It is important to obtain early serial tracings to observe the various ECG changes in pulmonary embolism.
7. $S_1Q_3T_3$ pattern (S wave in lead I, Q wave in lead III, inverted T wave in lead III). This is a "classic" combination of ECG findings that may be found in pulmonary embolism.

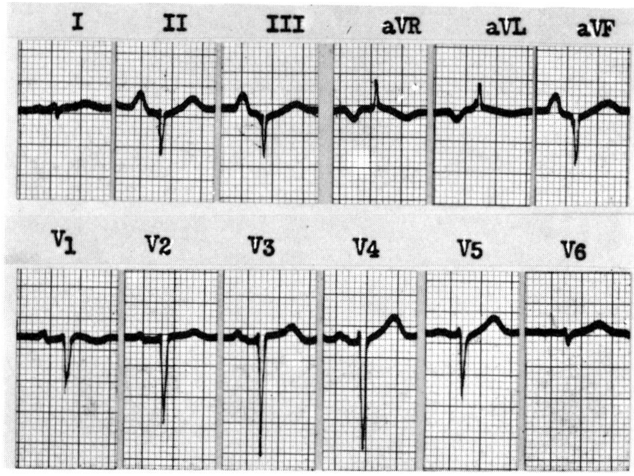

FIG 9–15.
ECG changes in chronic obstructive pulmonary disease (COPD). Note the large prominent P waves in *II, III, aVF* (P pulmonale), extreme right axis deviation (RAD) ($-100°$), poor R wave progression, and low voltage in the limb leads.

CHRONIC OBSTRUCTIVE PULMONARY DISEASE (COPD)

In COPD, a strain is placed on the right atrium and right ventricle as well as a shift of the position of the heart occurring inside the chest. The ECG features of COPD include the following:

1. *P nulmonale:* tall peaked P wave in leads II, III, aVF.
2. *RVH:* tall R wave in V_1; depressed ST segments and inverted T waves in chest leads V_1, V_2; etc. (see p. 117).
3. *RAD:* axis between $+90°$ and $+180°$; *extreme RAD:* axis between $+180°$ and $-90°$.
4. *Poor R wave progression* (PRWP, see Fig 2–7,*C*): In chronic obstructive lung disease, the right ventricle rotates anteriorly while the left ventricle rotates posteriorly (clockwise rotation viewed from below). This rotation of the heart causes all six chest leads to record low R waves and deep S waves. This pattern of PRWP may be mistaken for anterior myocardial infarction.
5. *Low voltage of QRS complexes in the limb leads:* QRS height less than 5 mm. This results from the hyperinflated lungs, which increases the distance between the heart and the recording electrodes.
6. *Supraventricular arrhythmias:* most commonly APCs and MAT.

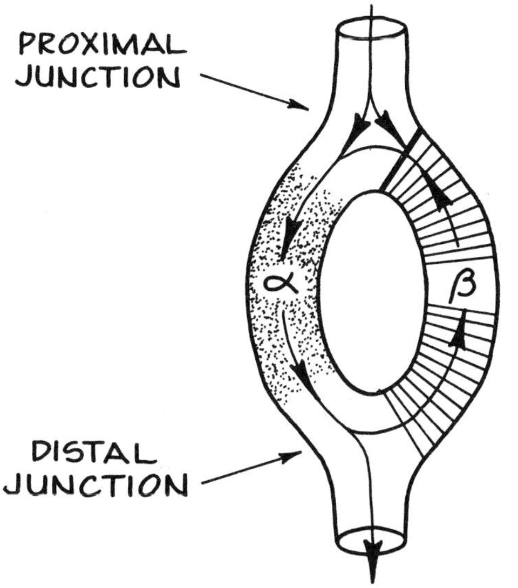

FIG 9–16.
Reentry circuit. It is composed of two pathways (α and β), which are joined at both ends. Each pathway possesses a different rate of conduction and a different refractory period. See text.

REENTRY

Reentry is the mechanism frequently postulated to cause atrial and ventricular tachyarrhythmias (rapid arrhythmias). It involves two independent pathways designated α (alpha) and β (beta), which are joined at their proximal and distal ends to form a closed loop. Each pathway has a different rate of conduction and a different refractory period (time required to fully repolarize). The α pathway has a *slower* rate of conduction and a *shorter* refractory period. The β pathway has a *faster* rate of conduction and a *longer* refractory period.

When an impulse enters the proximal junction of a reentry circuit, it travels antegrade (forward) through the α pathway because of its *shorter* refractory period. Conduction through the β pathway is blocked because of its *longer* refractory period. After the impulse travels through the α pathway to the distal junction, it *exits* through the distal junction as well as *enters* the distal end of the β pathway, which is no longer refractory at this time. The impulse travels retrograde (backward) in the β pathway to the proximal junction where it *reenters* and travels antegrade through the α pathway again. This reentry circuit or loop perpetuates itself until abolished.

A reentry circuit may occur at any site in the heart: SA node, atria, AV junction, or in the ventricles.

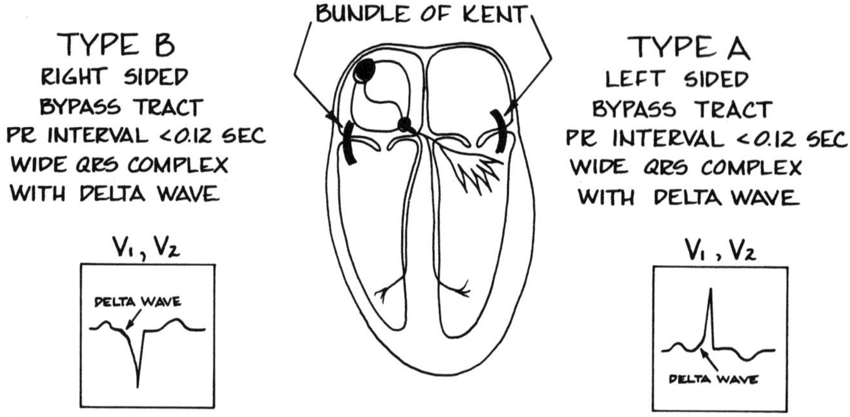

FIG 9–17.
WPW syndrome. *Type A* indicates a left-sided bypass tract with predominantly positive QRS complexes in leads V_1, V_2. *Type B* indicates a right-sided bypass tract with predominantly negative QRS complexes in leads V_1, V_2. It should be noted that these two classifications are not always accurate in localizing the bypass tracts.

PREEXCITATION SYNDROMES

Wolff-Parkinson-White (WPW) Syndrome

Preexcitation is abnormal *early* excitation of the ventricles. Preexcitation occurs through *accessory* conducting fibers that activate the ventricles early. This causes ventricular depolarization (QRS complex) to begin earlier than if an impulse had traveled through the normal AV conducting system and thus avoids the "delay" in the AV node.

The WPW syndrome is one type of preexcitation phenomenon whereby impulses are conducted from the atria to the ventricles through an *accessory* bypass tract called the *bundle of Kent* (above figure). Ventricular depolarization (QRS complex) begins early (preexcitation) through the bundle of Kent. This causes shortening of the P-R interval and an abnormal *initial* QRS deflection termed "delta wave," which *widens* the QRS complex. The remainder of ventricular depolarization occurs via normal conduction through the AV node, which *fuses* with the early depolarization impulse from the bypass tract (fusion beat).

The ECG manifestations of WPW syndrome include the following:

1. Short P-R interval: less than 0.12 second.
2. Wide QRS complex caused by a "delta" wave. The delta wave is the initial slurring of the QRS complex, which represents the premature activation of the ventricles from the bypass tract.

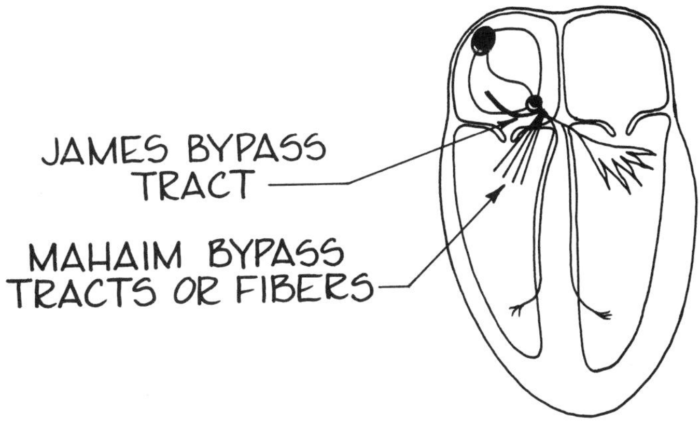

FIG 9–18.
Two types of preexcitation syndromes. (1), Lown-Ganong-Levine (LGL), which utilizes the James bypass tract, and (2), the Mahaim bypass tract. In the LGL syndrome, the James tract "preexcites" the lower area of the AV node or directly to the bundle of His, avoiding the "delay area" in the AV node, resulting in a short P-R and normal QRS. Mahaim fibers "preexcite" this right ventricle after the impulse has passed through the AV node, resulting in a normal P-R and wide QRS.

PREEXCITATION SYNDROMES

Lown-Ganong-Levine Syndrome
Mahaim Tracts

Two other types of *preexcitation* syndromes are the Lown-Ganong-Levine (LGL) syndrome and the Mahaim bypass tract syndrome. Both cause early depolarization of the ventricles (preexcitation).

The LGL syndrome utilizes an accessory tract (James bypass tract), which joins the atrium directly to the bundle of His. The James tract bypasses the "delay area" in the AV node so that conduction proceeds *earlier* and *unchanged* through the ventricles. There is shortening of the P-R interval (P-R less than 0.12 second) with a normal QRS complex and no delta wave.

The Mahaim *accessory* tracts or fibers have been shown to join the bundle of His directly to the right ventricle. The delay in the AV node is preserved, which results in a normal P-R interval. However, early excitation of the right ventricle through the Mahaim tracts results in a wide QRS complex resembling LBBB. No delta wave is present.

In summary, note the following:

1. LGL syndrome (James bypass tract): short P-R interval; no delta wave; normal QRS complex.
2. Mahaim bypass tract: normal P-R interval; no delta wave; wide QRS complex resembling LBBB.

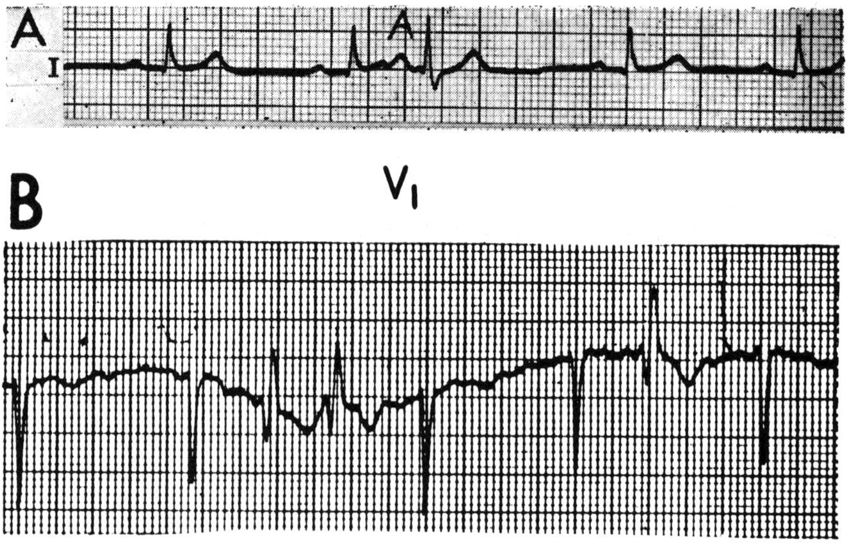

FIG 9–19.

A, APC displaying aberrant ventricular conduction. The early atrial impulse *(A)* conducts to the ventricles when the ventricles have not fully repolarized. Note the short R-R cycle (with the aberrant QRS) preceded by a long R-R cycle. This results in a wide QRS complex from aberrant ventricular conduction. **B,** Ashman beats. During atrial fibrillation, the earlier supraventricular impulses are aberrantly conducted in the ventricles, resulting in wide QRS complexes. Note the long-short intervals preceding the Ashman beats.

ABERRANT VENTRICULAR CONDUCTION

Ashman Phenomenon

Aberrant ventricular conduction refers to abnormal depolarization of the ventricles. This occurs when a supraventricular impulse reaches the ventricles before the ventricles are fully repolarized. Those ventricular fibers that are not fully repolarized are *refractory* to activation. A supraventricular impulse entering at this time depolarizes the ventricles in an abnormal fashion (Fig 9–19,*A*).

The ECG records aberrant ventricular conduction as a bizarre, wide QRS complex that is similar in configuration to the QRS complex of a ventricular ectopic beat. It is important to differentiate the wide QRS complex of *aberrant ventricular conduction* (initiated from a supraventricular impulse) from the wide QRS complex of a *ventricular ectopic impulse* (initiated from a ventricular focus). The clinical implication of the latter can be more serious than the former.

Ashman phenomenon is a form of aberrant ventricular conduction that occurs during atrial fibrillation when a long R-R interval is followed by a short R-R interval (see Fig 5–15). Importantly, the Ashman phenomenon (wide QRS complex) denotes a supraventricular impulse during atrial fibrillation associated with aberrant ventricular conduction and should not be mistaken for a ventricular ectopic beat (Fig 9–19,*B*).

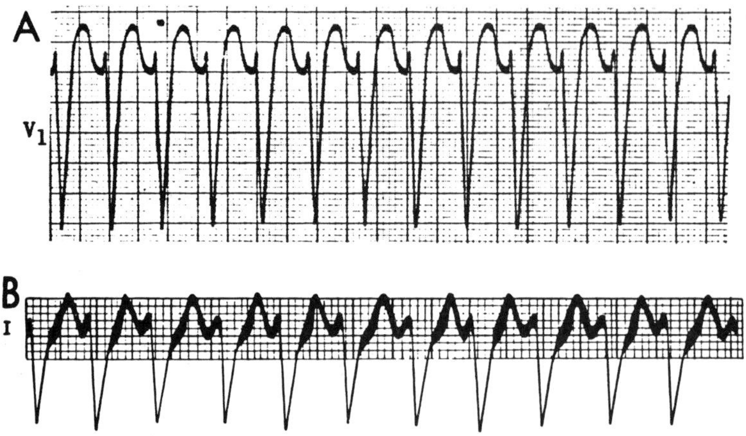

FIG 9–20.
A, *supraventricular tachycardia* at a rate of 175 beats/min in a patient with preexisting left bundle branch block (LBBB). Note its similarity to ventricular tachycardia. **B,** ventricular tachycardia at a rate of 175 beats/min. Note the wide QRS complexes are similar to **A.**

DIFFERENTIAL DIAGNOSIS OF WIDE QRS COMPLEX TACHYCARDIAS

Awareness that a wide QRS complex tachycardia is not necessarily due to ventricular tachycardia is clinically important. If the site of origin of the tachycardia is supraventricular, the wide QRS complexes may represent (1) *aberrant ventricular conduction*, (2) *bundle branch block*, or (3) *preexcitation of the ventricles*. If the site of origin of the wide QRS tachycardia is ventricular, the cause is *ventricular tachycardia*, which may progress to ventricular fibrillation and death. Differentiating ventricular tachycardia from *supraventricular tachycardia with aberration* has been reviewed by Wellens et al.* The ECG findings suggestive of *ventricular tachycardia* include:

1. QRS duration greater than 0.14 second.
2. LAD greater than $-30°$.
3. AV dissociation with fusion beats (FB) and sinus capture beats.
4. QRS morphologies in lead V_1 of RS 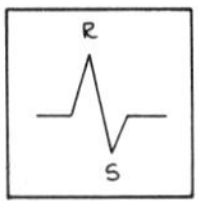

, RSr′ 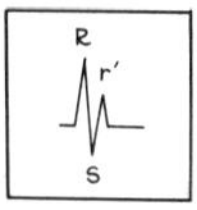

.
5. QRS morphologies in lead V_6 of qR 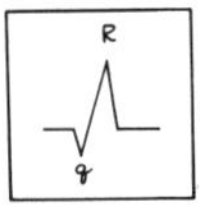

, QS 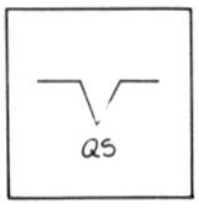

, R:S ratio less than one 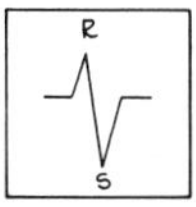

.

The ECG findings suggestive of *supraventricular tachycardia with aberrant ventricular conduction* include the following:

1. QRS duration less than 0.14 second.
2. QRS morphology in lead V_1 of rsR′ 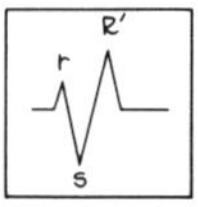

.

Note: In patients with preexcitation syndrome (bypass tract) or bundle branch block, differentiation is not possible using these criteria.

---

*Wellens HJJ, et al: The value of the electrocardiogram in the differential diagnosis of a tachycardia with a widened QRS complex. *Am J Med* 1978; 64:27–32.

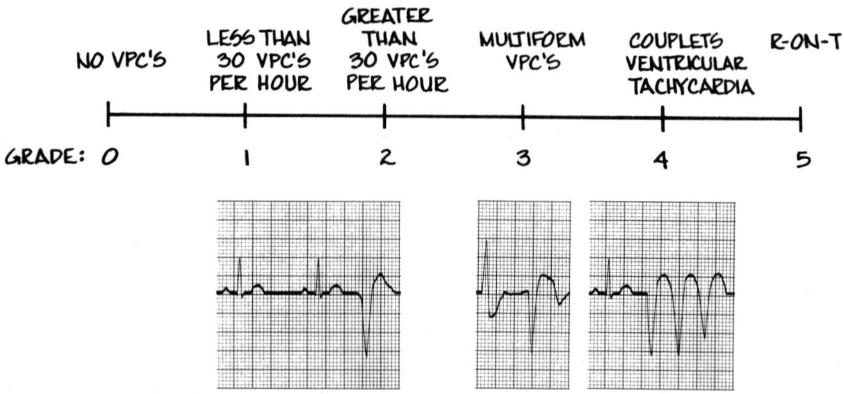

FIG 9–21.
Lown's grading system for ventricular ectopy.

GRADING SYSTEM FOR VENTRICULAR ECTOPY

Different grades of ventricular ectopic impulses have been suggested by Lown and Graboys* and are listed sequentially from less to more severe grades:

Grade

- 0: No VPCs
- I: Less than 30 VPCs per hour
  - a. Less than one VPC per minute
  - b. Greater than one VPC per minute
- II: Greater than 30 VPCs per hour
- III: Multiform VPCs
- IV: a. Couplets
  - b. Greater than two consecutive VPCs, runs of paroxysmal ventricular tachycardia.
- V: R-on-T phenomenon (see Fig 5–21, p. 67)

Prognosis and therapy of ventricular arrhythmias ultimately depends on the clinical situation. For further reading, another classification has been suggested by Myerburg et al.†

---

*Lown B, Graboys T.: Management of patients with malignant ventricular arrhythmias. *Am J Cardiol* 1977; 39:910–918.

†Myerburg RJ et al: Classification of ventricular arrhythmias based on parallel hierarchies of frequency and form. *Am J Cardiol* 1984; 54:1355–1358.

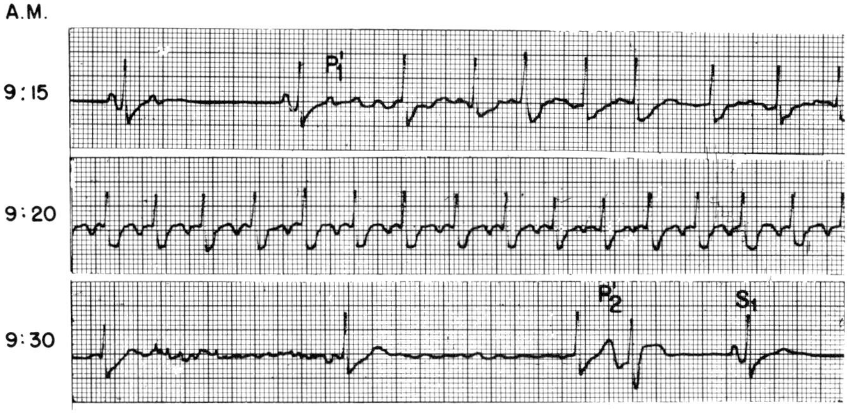

FIG 9–22.
Sick sinus syndrome. Note the alternating tachycardia and bradycardia. *Strip 1 (9:15),* sudden onset of atrial fibrillation after APC *(P'_1).* *Strip 2 (9:20),* atrial flutter with 2:1 block. *Strip 3 (9:30),* atrial fibrillation with slow escape rhythm followed by APC *(P'_2)* and sinus beat *(S_1).*

SICK SINUS SYNDROME

Sick sinus syndrome, otherwise known as "bradycardia-tachycardia" syndrome, encompasses a variety of arrhythmias. As the name implies, there is sinus node dysfunction. However, arrhythmias also occur in the atria, AV junction, and ventricular conducting system. Sick sinus syndrome usually results from degeneration or fibrosis in the SA node and elsewhere in the conducting system of the heart.

The arrhythmias of sick sinus syndrome include bradyarrhythmias (slow arrhythmias), sinus pause, sinus arrest, marked sinus bradycardia or junctional bradycardia that may alternate with various tachyarrhythmias (rapid arrhythmias), atrial fibrillation, atrial flutter, and PAT, thus popularizing the term "brady-tachy" syndrome.

Symptoms from sick sinus syndrome are due to the very slow or very fast heart rhythms and include palpitations, dizziness, and fainting episodes (syncope). The most effective treatment is insertion of a pacemaker for the bradyarrhythmias. Drugs may be used to treat the tachyarrhythmias once a pacemaker has been inserted.

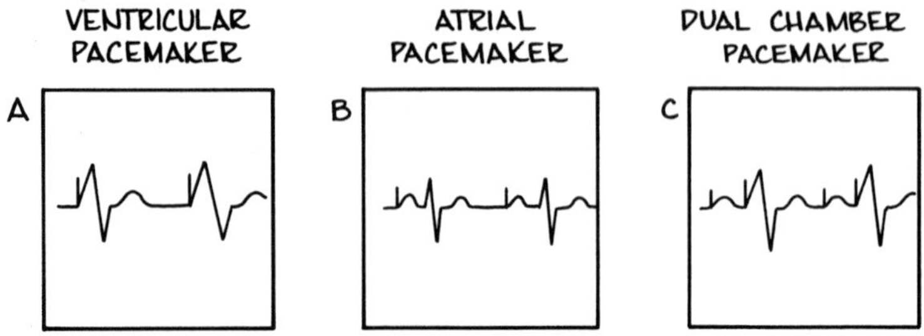

FIG 9–23.
ECG pacemaker patterns. **A,** *ventricular pacemaker.* **B,** *atrial pacemaker.* **C,** *dual chamber pacemaker* demonstrating paced atrial activation, then paced ventricular activation.

ARTIFICIAL PACEMAKER RHYTHMS

Pacemakers are artificial devices comprised of a battery-powered generator and wire electrodes that are used to pace the heart. The wire electrode is placed in the atrium or ventricle or both chambers and transmits impulses between the generator and heart. If the electrode is placed in the right atrium and an impulse is delivered, the ECG records a straight vertical line called pacemaker spike, which is followed by a wide P wave (from abnormal atrial depolarization). If the electrode is placed in the right ventricle and an impulse is delivered, the ECG records a pacemaker spike followed by a wide QRS complex. When the electrode is in the right ventricle, the paced QRS complex resembles a LBBB pattern, because activation begins in the right ventricle and terminates in the left ventricle, simulating LBBB.

Sophisticated dual-chamber pacemakers have been developed that use both atrial and ventricular electrodes to activate first the atria and then the ventricles. This sequence of activation simulates the normal AV conduction sequence and provides the advantage of an "atrial kick." Depending on the particular model and programming of the dual-chamber pacemaker, the ECG may show neither, either, or both atrial and ventricular pacemaker functions. Note that the atrial or ventricular pacemaker spikes may not be visible in every lead and may vary in height in the different limb and chest leads.

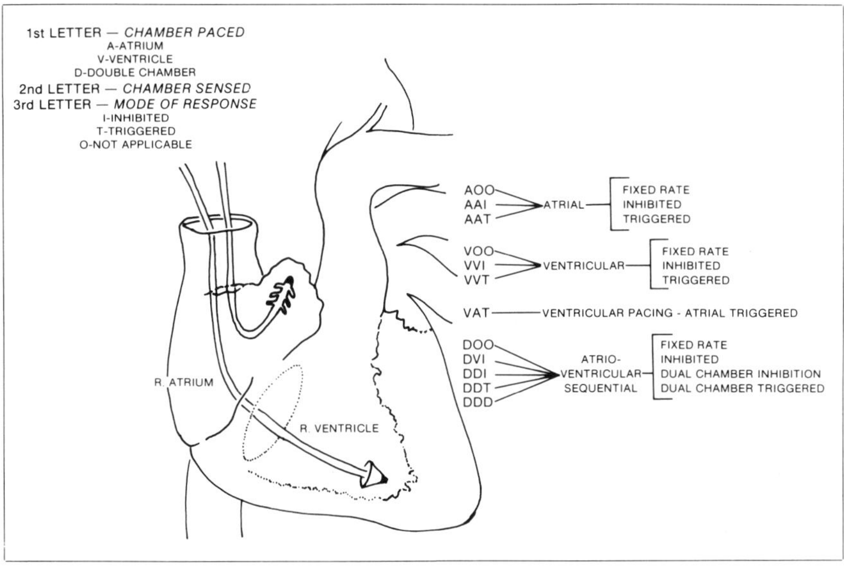

FIG 9–24.
The code system of pacemakers using the first three positions of the code.

PACEMAKER TERMINOLOGY

In order to diagnose pacemaker malfunction, the type and model of the pacemaker generator, as well as the site or sites of the wire electrodes, should be known. A coding system of the different types of pacemaker has been devised. The code consists of a five-letter designation for each pacemaker (see Table 3 and Fig 9–24):

1. The first letter refers to the chamber that is paced, i.e., the heart chamber that is stimulated. *A* refers to atrium, *V* to ventricle, *D* to both chambers.
2. The second letter refers to the heart chamber that is sensed. The same letters (*A*, *V*, and *D*) are used as for the first position.
3. The third letter refers to the mode of response—pacemaker's response to sensed events. *I* refers to inhibition, *T* refers to triggering of the output circuit, and *D* is used to indicate both functions.
4. The fourth letter refers to the programmable functions—capability of altering pacemaker functions noninvasively.
5. The fifth letter refers to special tachyarrhythmia functions—specific antitachycardia features. (See reference text for more in-depth review).

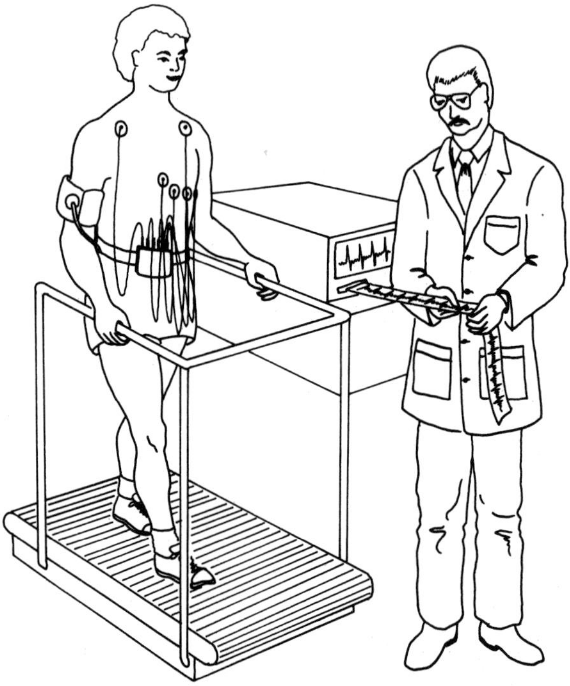

FIG 9–25.
Exercise treadmill testing.

EXERCISE TESTING

Exercise testing is an excellent noninvasive method for evaluating patients, diagnosing ischemic heart disease, assessing the patient's functional capacity, and selecting patients for cardiac catheterization. *"Low-level"* exercise testing is useful for predicting future cardiac events as well as for assessing and reassuring patients after acute myocardial infarction, coronary artery bypass surgery, and coronary angioplasty. The combination of exercise testing with nuclear imaging increases the accuracy of the test (see reference text).

Exercise according to specific "staged" protocols (such as Bruce protocol, Table 4) is performed on a treadmill or bicycle ergometer. The work load on a treadmill is increased in stages by increasing the speed and incline at 3-minute intervals. Serial ECGs and blood pressure recordings are taken at each stage, and continuous ECG monitoring is performed throughout the test in the presence of qualified personnel with emergency equipment.

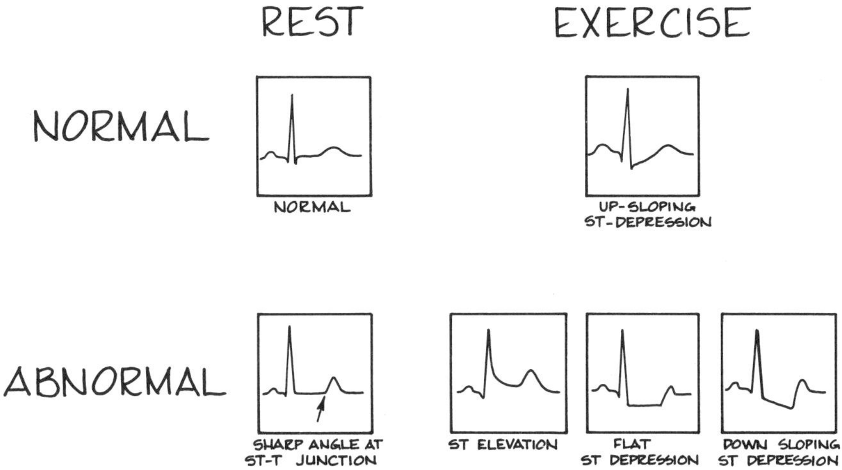

FIG 9–26.
The *normal* and *abnormal* changes in configuration of the ST segment at *rest* and during *exercise.* Note the flat, horizontal ST in the abnormal rest ECG.

ECG CHANGES DURING EXERCISE TESTING

The *normal* ECG response to exercise is as follows:

1. Increase in heart rate
2. Increase in P wave amplitude
3. Shortening of the P-R and Q-T intervals
4. Decrease in the R wave amplitude
5. Shift of the QRS axis to the right
6. Depressed J point with upsloping ST segment
7. Variable T wave changes

An *abnormal, positive* ECG response to exercise includes the following:

1. Depressed J point with *horizontal* or *downsloping* ST depression greater than 1 mm, with or without angina. The *greater the ST depression,* the *earlier the onset* of ST depression (stage I or stage II), and the *longer the duration* of ST depression are important diagnostic criteria
2. ST elevation greater than 1 mm
3. Increase in the R wave amplitude
4. Inversion of U waves
5. Significant arrhythmias

False positive exercise tests may occur with the following:

1. Digitalis
2. Hypokalemia
3. Ventricular hypertrophy
4. Bundle branch block
5. Preexcitation syndromes (WPW)
6. Mitral valve prolapse
7. Female sex

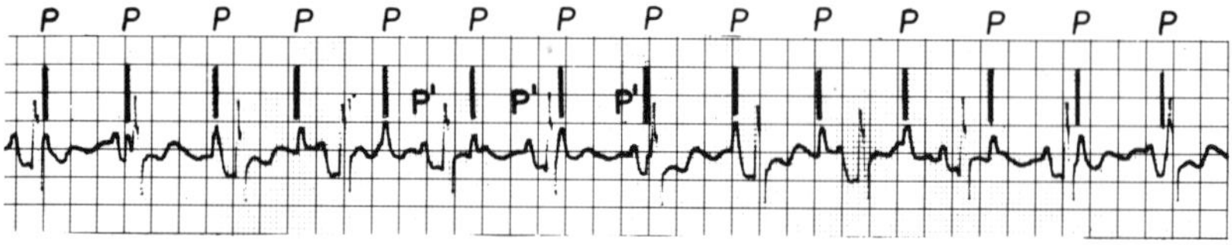

FIG 9–27.
ECG after cardiac transplantation. The *P′* represents atrial activity of the new donor heart, which controls the ventricles. The second parasystolic nonconducting P waves *(P)* represent activity from the recipient's remnant SA node. These P waves beat independently of the donor rhythm.

CARDIAC TRANSPLANTATION ECG CHANGES

After *cardiac transplantation* of a normal donor heart into a recipient, the rhythm is usually sinus with normal P-R and QRS durations and normal QRS axis. There may be nonspecific ST and T changes because of drug or metabolic effects following surgery. Often a second parasystolic P wave is recorded that beats independently of the donor heart rhythm. This independent atrial rhythm is produced by the recipient's native SA node, which remains in a ring of the recipient's atrium. The sinus impulses from this remnant SA node are unable to conduct to the new donor heart, and with time, its activity extinguishes itself.

If rejection to the donor heart occurs, ECG changes include the following:

1. Decrease in QRS voltage
2. Rightward shift of the QRS axis
3. Right bundle branch block (RBBB)
4. Prolongation of the P-R interval
5. Supraventricular arrhythmias (APCs, atrial tachycardia with block, atrial fibrillation, junctional rhythm)
6. Nonspecific ST and T changes
7. VPCs

If the rejection process is successfully treated, the ECG reverts to normal.

PEARLS

1. Wide QRS tachycardia caused by *ventricular aberration* may manifest three or more different QRS configurations. In ventricular tachycardia, the QRS morphologies rarely manifest more than two different configurations.

2. Wide QRS tachycardia may be due to preexisting bundle branch block. Comparison with previous and subsequent ECGs is necessary for this diagnosis.

3. A wide QRS tachycardia that is very rapid (greater than 220 beats/min) and irregularly irregular suggests atrial fibrillation that is conducting impulses through an accessory bypass tract to the ventricles (WPW syndrome). This is often mistaken for ventricular tachycardia.

4. The ECG combination of acute *anterior* and/or *inferior* myocardial infarction, injury, or ischemia raises the possibility of acute pulmonary embolism.

5. Nonspecific ST-T changes (repolarization changes) can occur in numerous situations: drinking ice water, after eating, hyperventilation, postural changes, fear, anxiety, emotional disturbances, drugs, electrolyte imbalances, pancreatitis, shock, gallbladder disease, stroke, acute abdomen, and metabolic and endocrine abnormalities.

6. A subtle but important ECG finding in acute pericarditis is P-R segment depression in many of the leads.

7. During treatment of atrial fibrillation with digoxin, the acute regularization of the rhythm (junctional rhythm) suggests "Dig. toxicity."

10 / Illustrative ECGs

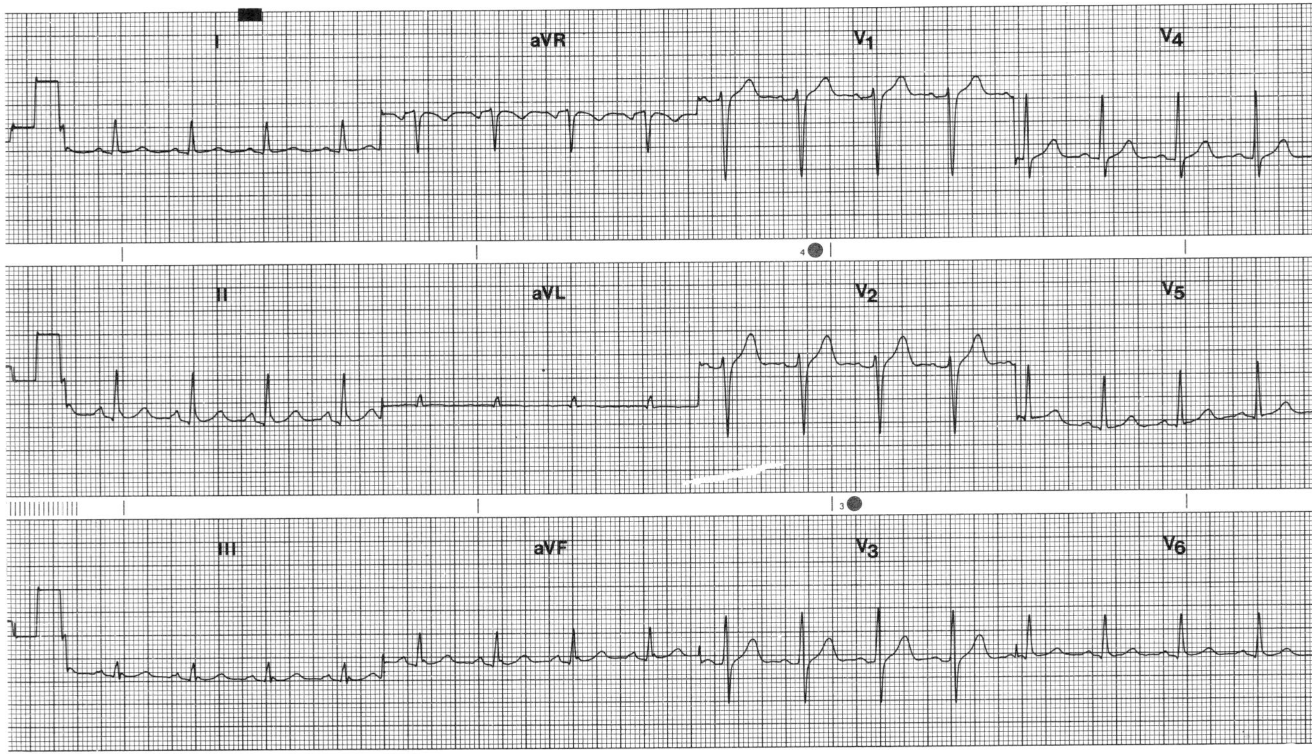

FIG 10–1.
43-year-old man. Normal 12-lead ECG. Normal sinus rhythm, rate 93 beats/min, QRS axis +50°, normal P-R and QRS intervals.

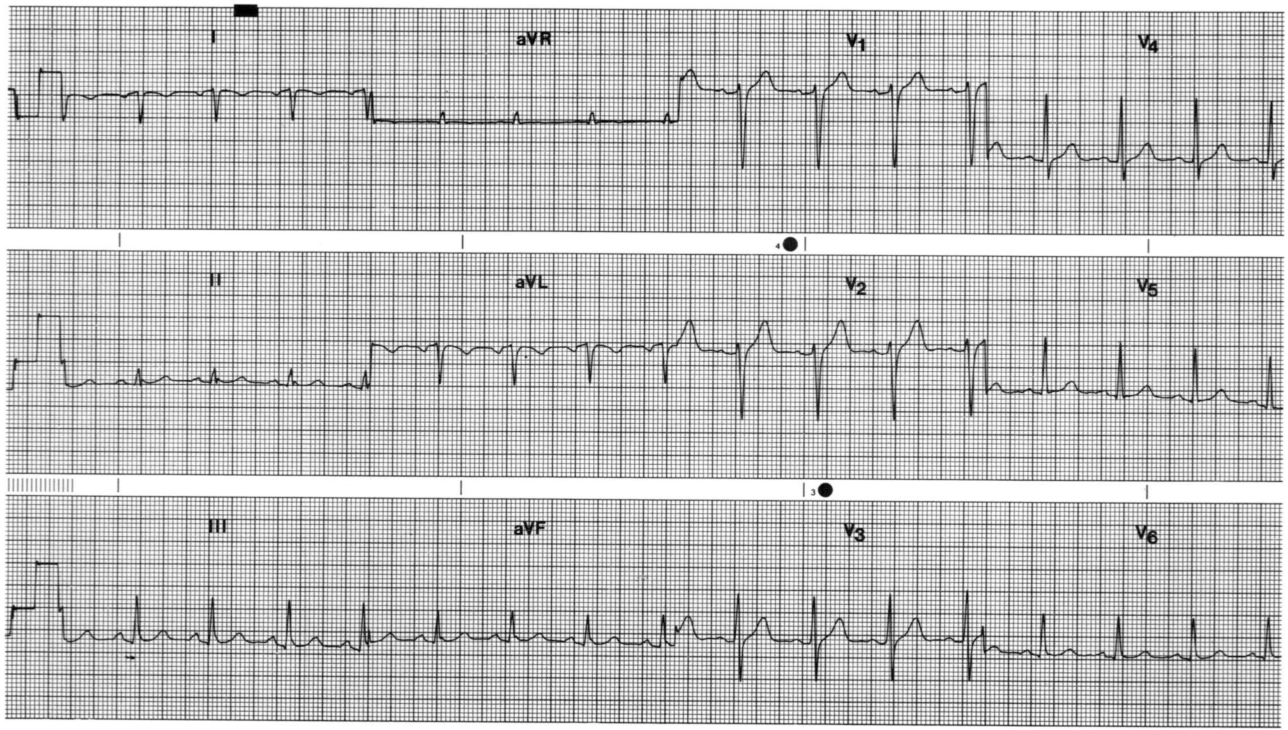

FIG 10–2.
Reversed electrodes. Same patient as in Fig 10–1. The right and left arm electrodes are reversed. Note the negative P. QRS, and T deflections in leads *I* and *aVL,* which alert the interpreter to the possibility of reversed electrodes. Lead *I* is mirror image of itself. Leads *aVR* and *aVL* are reversed. The chest leads remain the same.

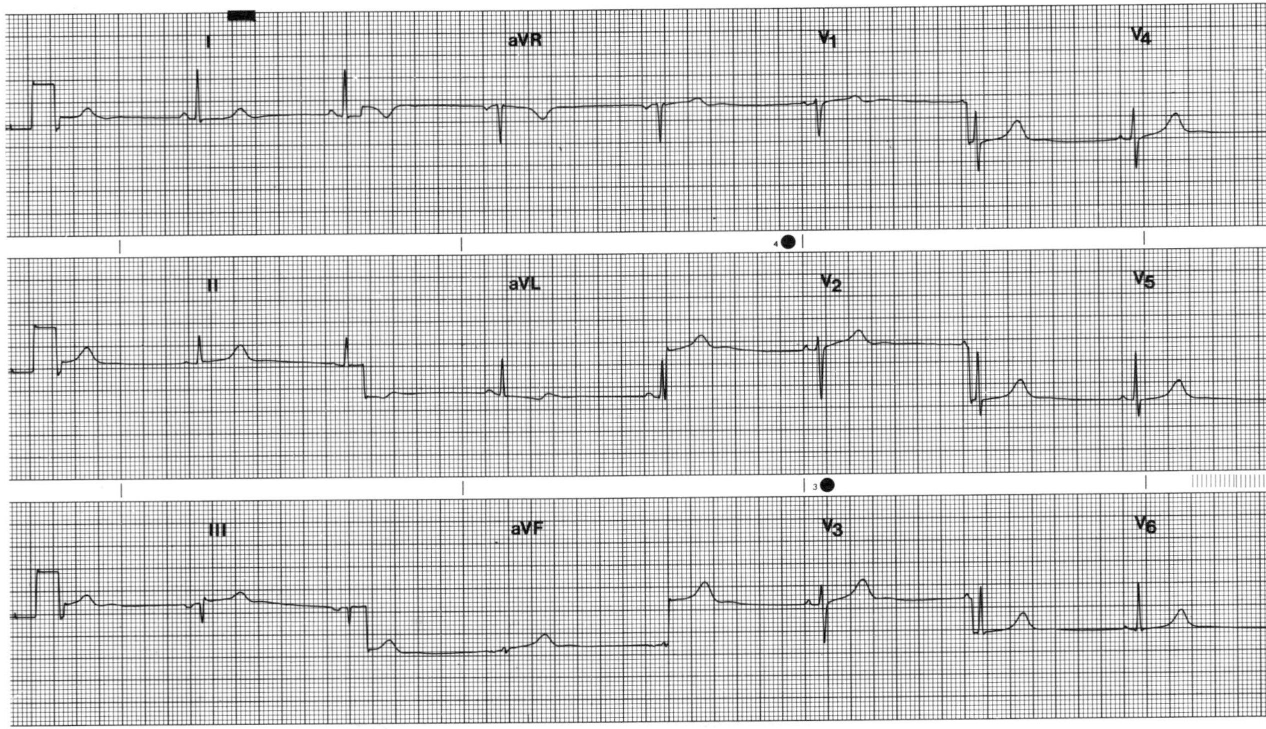

FIG 10–3.
Sinus bradycardia. 44-year-old woman. Rate 43 beats/min, QRS axis 0° (note the small, biphasic QRS deflection in lead *aVF*). The Q wave in lead *III* is a normal variant and may disappear with deep inspiration.

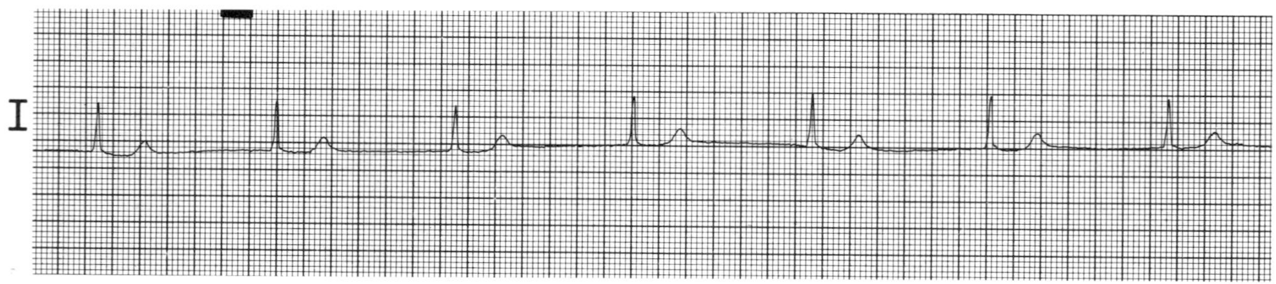

FIG 10–4.
Dig. toxicity. 70-year-old woman with coronary artery disease taking digoxin and diuretics. Lead *I*. Junctional rhythm, rate 47 beats/min. Note the absence of P waves, the junctional rhythm and scooped ST segments that are secondary to digoxin toxicity.

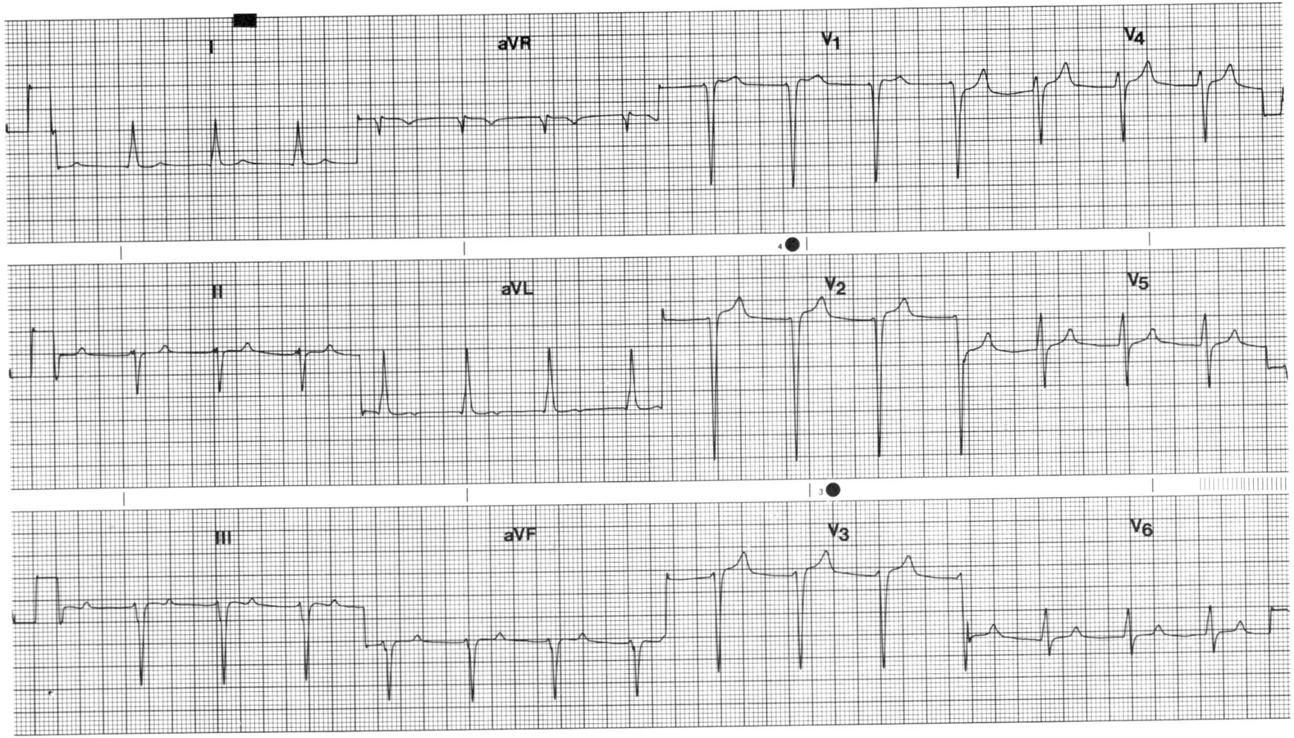

FIG 10–5.
Dig. toxicity. Accelerated junctional rhythm. 52-year-old man with renal failure, diabetes mellitus, and hypertension, who was taking digoxin. Rate 84 beats/min, left anterior fascicular block *(LAFB)*, and probable left ventricular hypertrophy *(LVH)*. Note the absence of P waves and regularity of the rhythm consistent with junctional rhythm. The marked left axis deviation *(LAD)* (QRS axis −60°); tall R waves in *I, aVL;* and small r waves in *II, III, aVF* confirm the diagnosis of LAFB. Also note the deep S wave in V_2 (32 mm) and tall R wave in *aVL* (14 mm) with repolarization changes and widened QRS duration (0.11 second), which are consistent with LVH. The poor R wave progression in leads V_1 through V_4 is probably secondary to LVH and LAFB rather than an old anterior myocardial infarction.

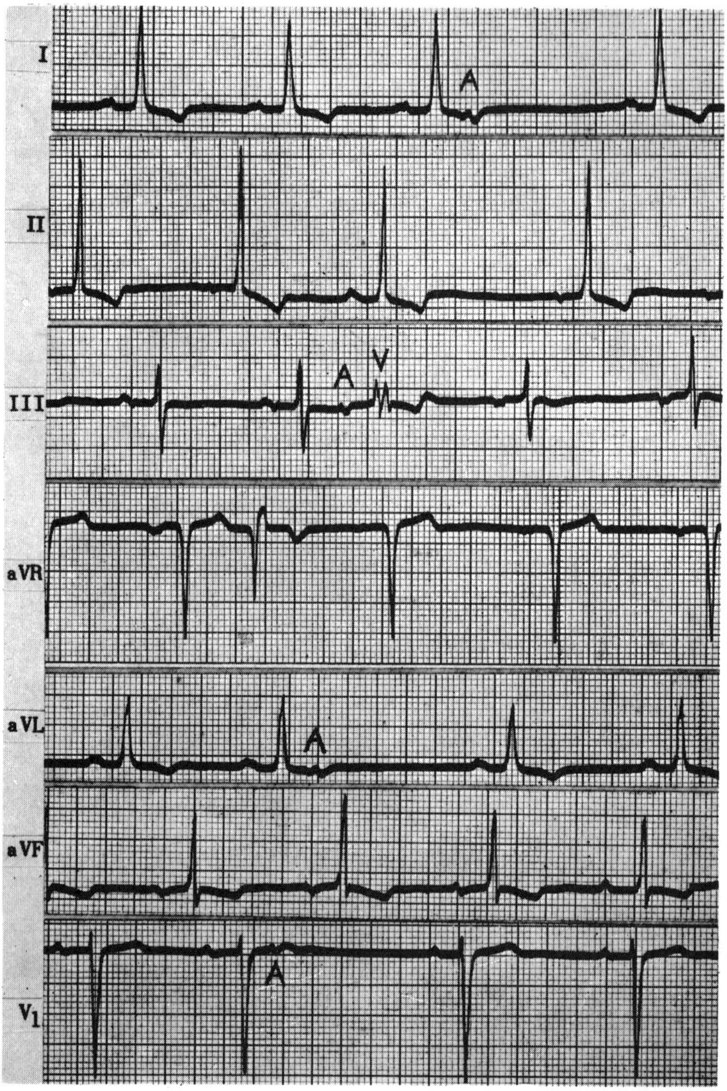

FIG 10–6.
Wandering atrial pacemaker, average rate 58 beats/min. Note the different P wave configurations, especially in *aVF.* Also note the atrial premature contractions (APCs) *(A)* that are *blocked* in *I, aVL,* and V_1. The APC *(A)* in *III* is followed by an aberrant QRS complex *(V).* Additionally, there are abnormal ST and T deflections in *I, II, aVL,* and *aVF* as well as prolonged P-R interval (0.22) consistent with "Dig. effect."

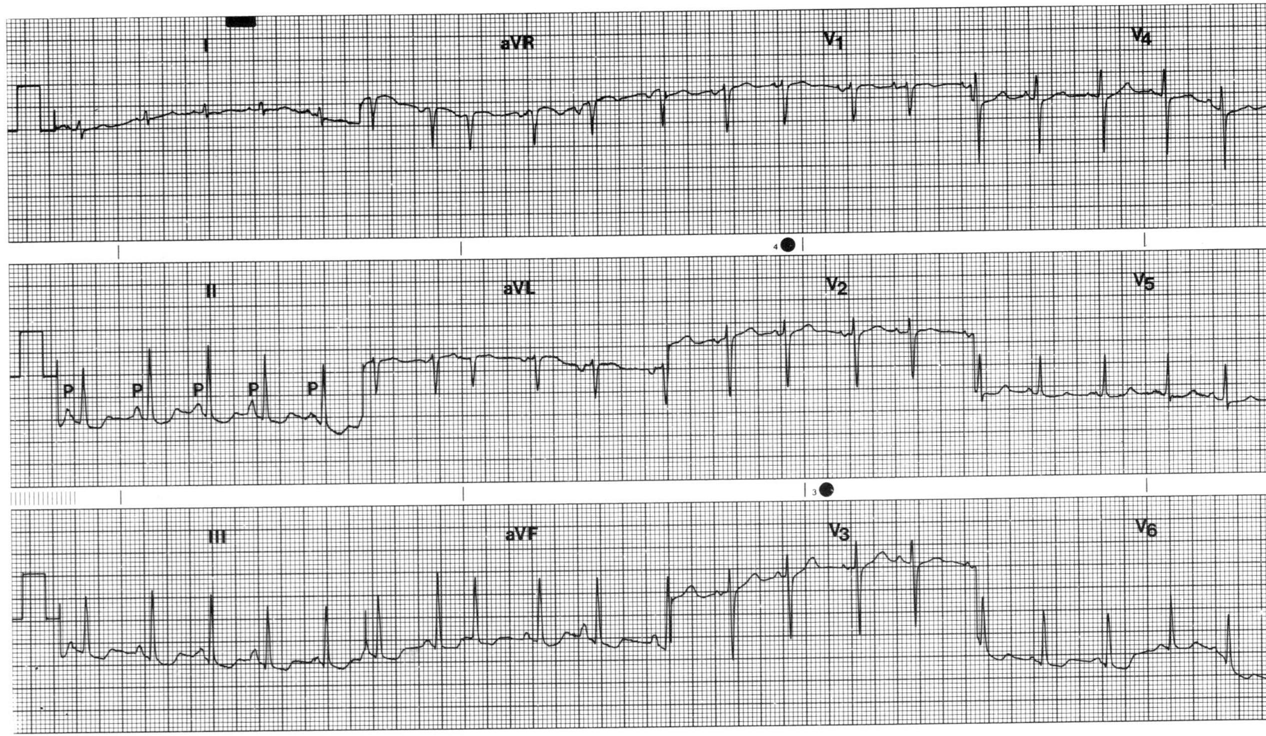

FIG 10–7.
Multifocal atrial tachycardia (MAT). 69-year-old woman with chronic obstructive pulmonary disease (COPD). Note the irregular rhythm with varying P-P intervals, varying P-R intervals and average rate of 115 beats/min. The tall, peaked P waves *(P)* in lead *II*, as well as leads *III* and *aVF*, indicate P pulmonale. Also note the rightward QRS axis (axis +80°) and poor R wave progression in leads V_1 through V_4 consistent with COPD.

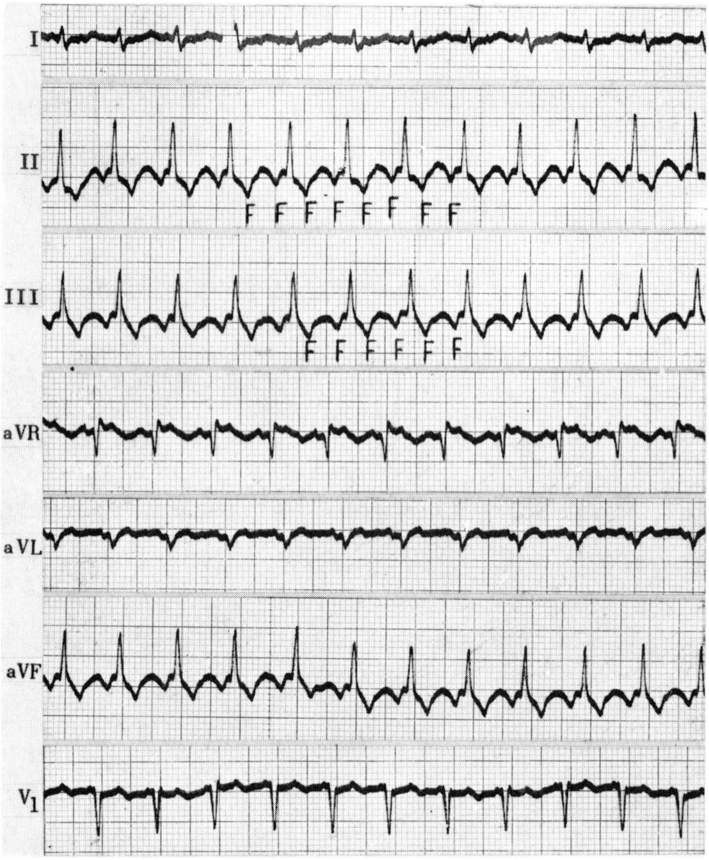

FIG 10–8.
Atrial flutter with 2:1 AV conduction. Atrial rate is 300 beats/min, and ventricular rate is 150 beats/min. The flutter *(F)* waves appear as a saw-tooth pattern and are best seen in the inferior leads *(II, III, aVF)*.

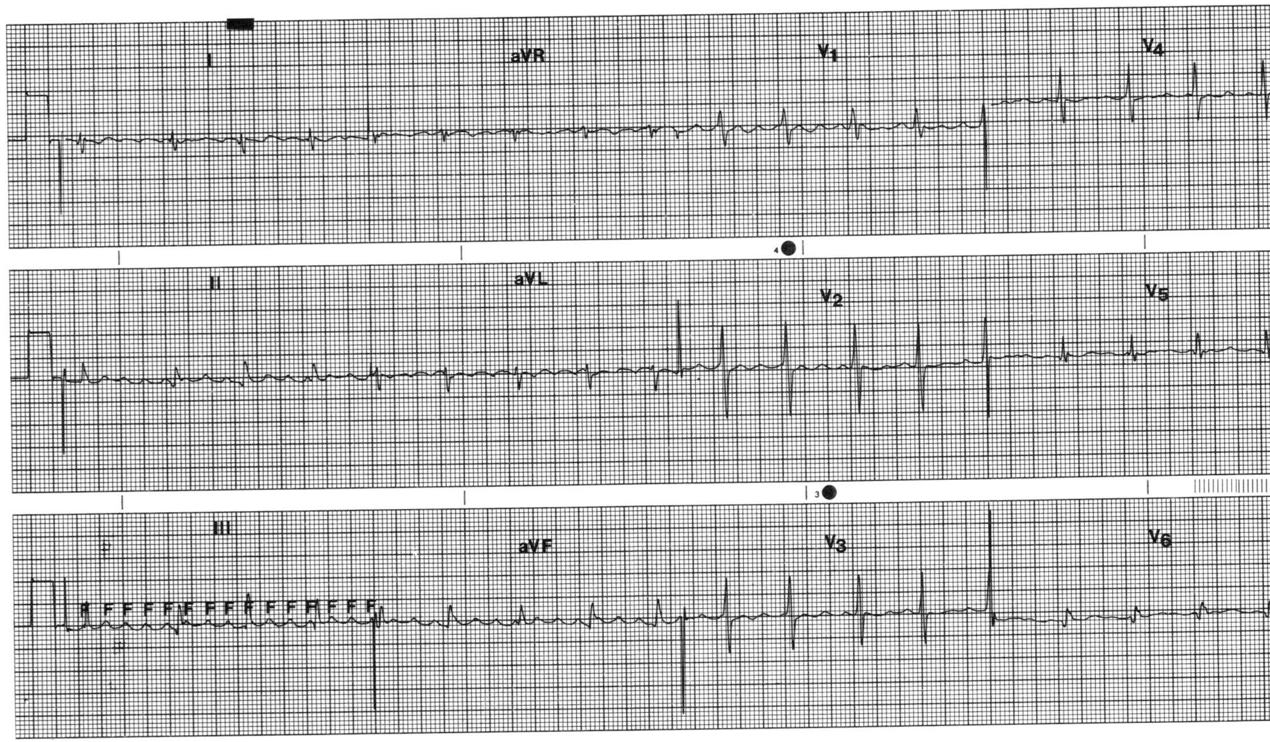

FIG 10–9.
50-year-old man with hypertension, coronary artery disease, and a previous old inferolateral myocardial infarction. Atrial flutter. The flutter *(F)* waves are best seen in the inferior leads *(II, III, aVF)* at a rate of 320 beats/min with varying 3:1 and 4:1 AV conduction resulting in a ventricular rate averaging 90–110 beats/min. The Q waves in *II, III, aVF,* and V_6 confirm the old inferolateral myocardial infarction. The tall R wave in V_1 suggests an associated posterior myocardial infarction.

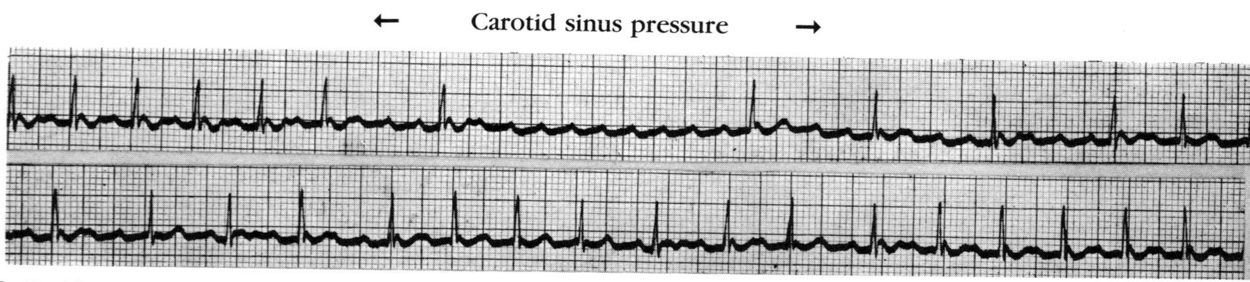

FIG 10–10.
Atrial flutter in a continuous strip of lead II. Note the initial 2:1 AV conduction blocking to 10:1 AV conduction with the application of carotid sinus pressure. When carotid sinus pressure was released, there was an irregular return to the original 2:1 conduction.

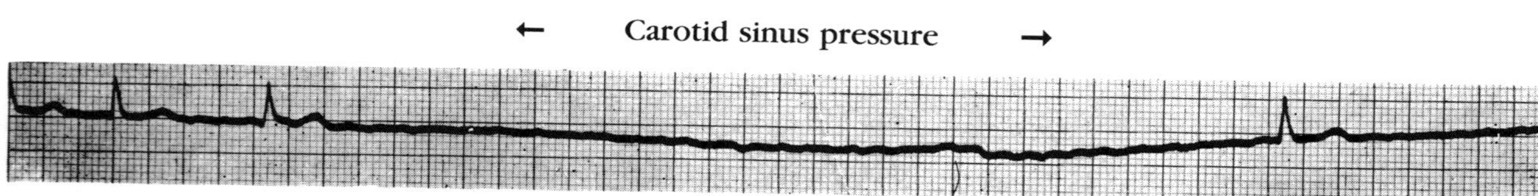

FIG 10–11.
Atrial fibrillation in lead II. Note the very marked effect of *carotid sinus pressure* resulting in a pause of 5.8 seconds.

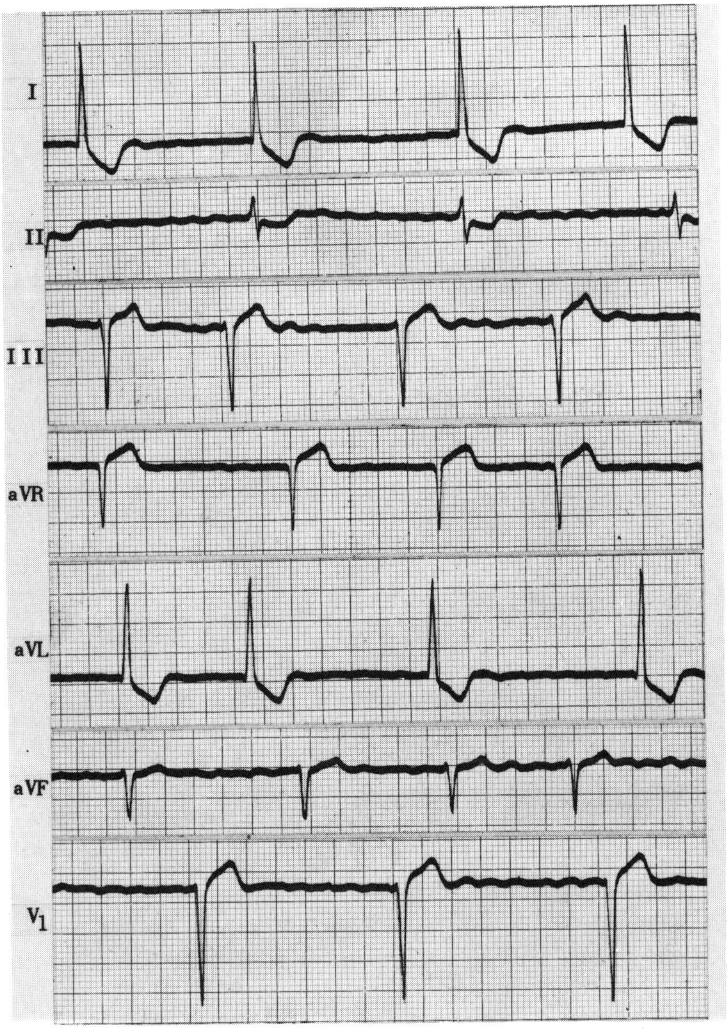

FIG 10–12.
Atrial fibrillation with a slow irregularly irregular ventricular rate of 42 to 70 beats/min. Note the undulating fibrillatory waves, varying in size and shape, which are best seen in leads *II, III, aVF,* and V_1. Also note the ST-T changes of "Dig. effect."

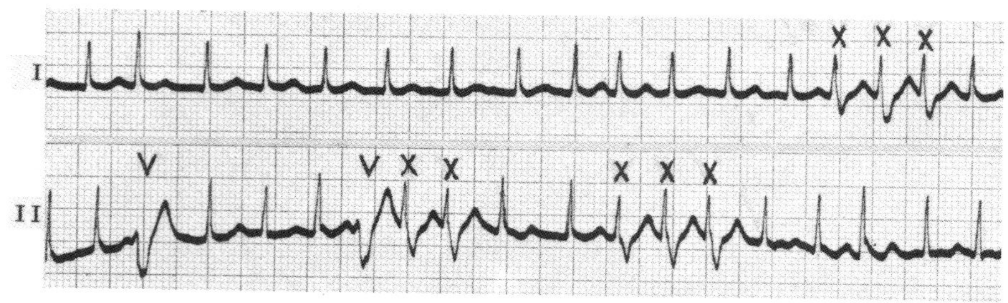

FIG 10–13.
Atrial fibrillation with Ashman beats. Note the rapid irregularly irregular ventricular response of around 150 beats/min. The wider QRS complexes *(X)* are Ashman beats and represent ventricular aberration, which is common in atrial fibrillation associated with a rapid ventricular response. The two widest QRS complexes *(V)* in lead *II* resemble ventricular premature contractions (VPCs), but are more likely to be a more pronounced degree of aberrant ventricular conduction (Ashman beats); these two beats have shorter coupling intervals and resemble RBBB with LAFB.

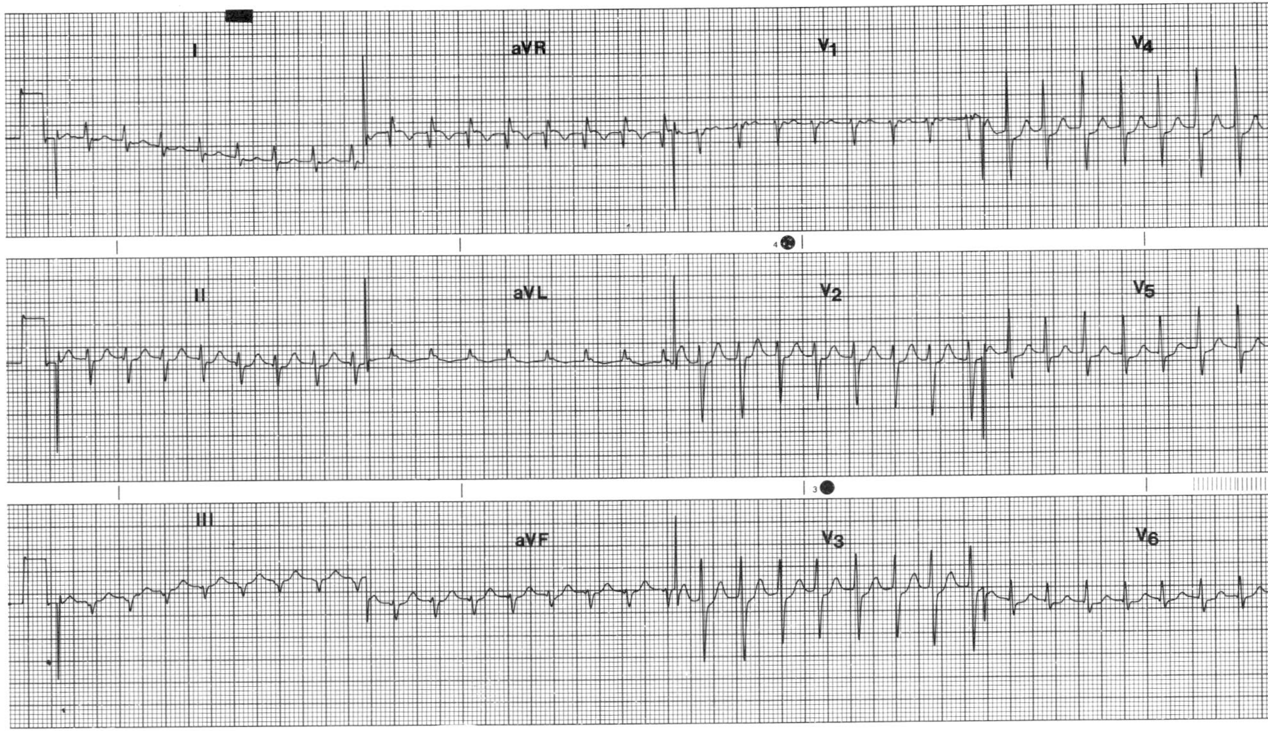

FIG 10–14.
Supraventricular tachycardia (SVT). 50-year-old man with a history of intermittent episodes of palpitations. Supraventricular tachycardia with narrow QRS complexes, rate of 190 beats/min, and left anterior fascicular block (LAFB). The mechanism of the tachycardia is most likely a reentry circuit in the AV junction (AV junctional reentrant tachycardia or PAT). Note in lead V_1 the retrograde P waves immediately following the QRS complexes. The marked left axis deviation (QRS axis −75°) is consistent with LAFB.

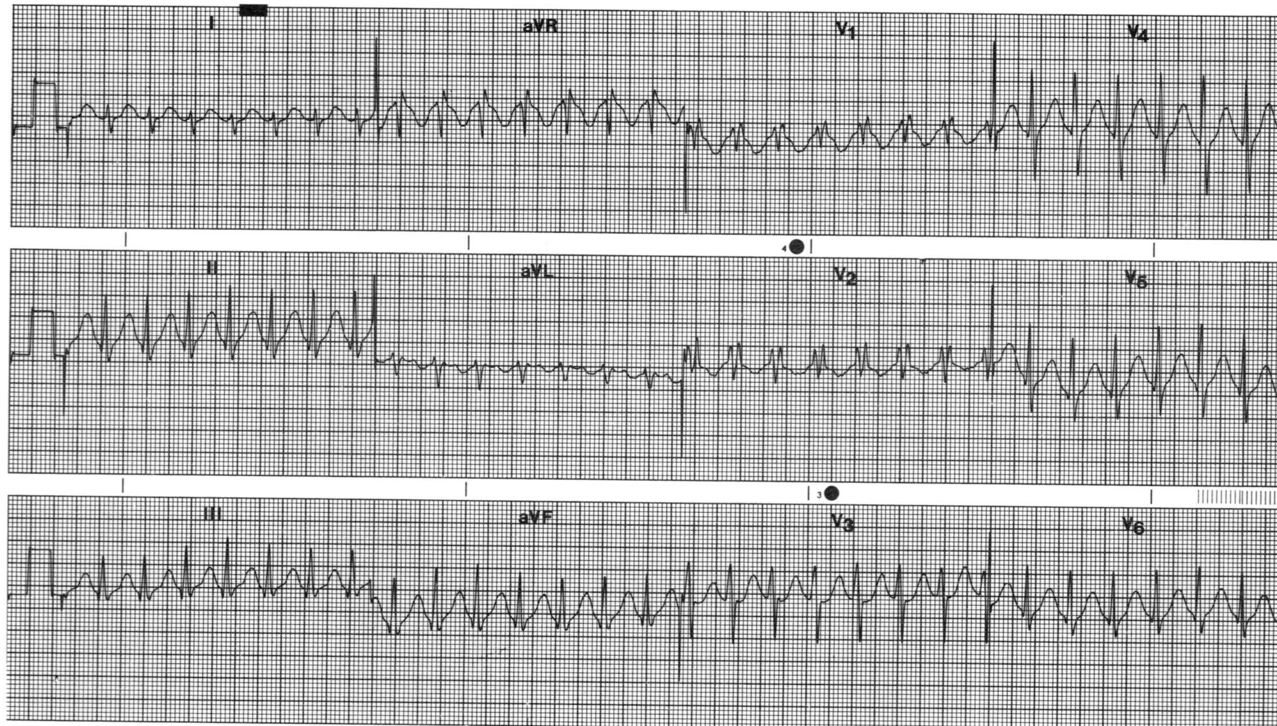

FIG 10–15.
22-year-old woman with an overdose from a tricyclic antidepressant. Supraventricular tachycardia, rate 170 beats/min, right axis deviation (RAD) (QRS axis +110°), and right bundle branch block (RBBB). Note the broad, abnormal T waves characteristic of tricyclic toxicity. Two days later, the rhythm returned to sinus, the RAD returned to normal, and the RBBB resolved corresponding to the decrease in tricyclic blood levels.

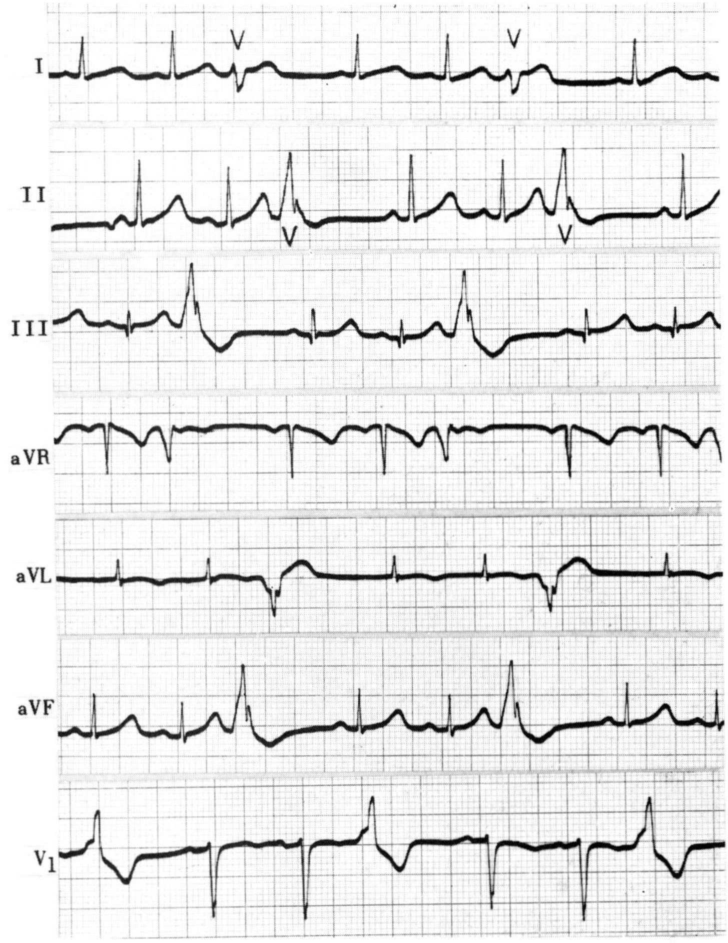

FIG 10–16.
Ventricular premature contractions (VPCs). The configuration of the VPCs *(V)* are identical in *each lead,* indicating a single ectopic focus. They occur regularly, after two normal beats *(trigeminy).* The coupling intervals are constant.

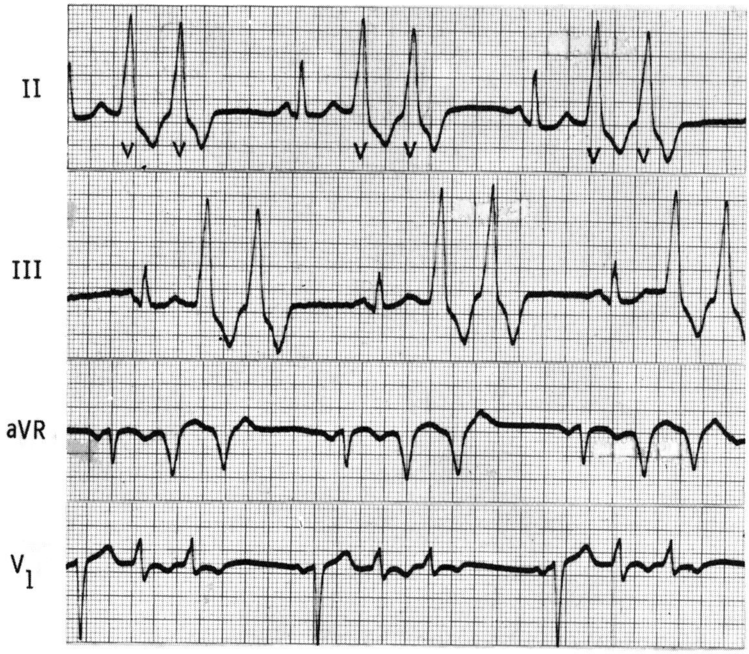

FIG 10–17.
Sinus rhythm with frequent ventricular premature contractions *(V)*. The rhythm is another form of *trigeminy* consisting of one sinus beat followed by two consecutive VPCs (couplets).

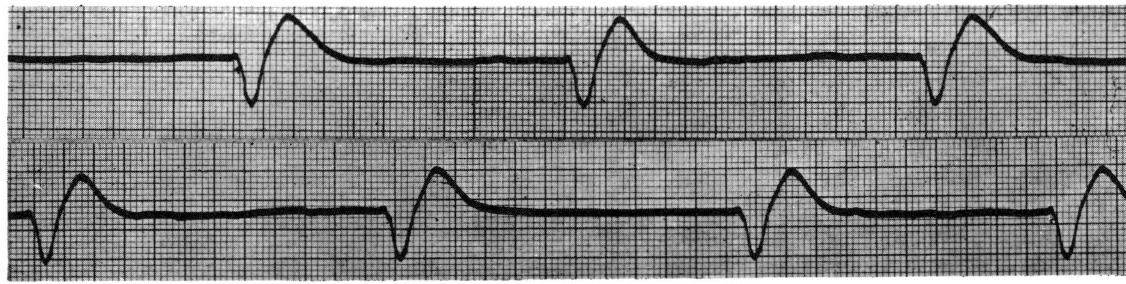

FIG 10–18.
Idioventricular rhythm, rate 27 beats/min in a dying patient. No atrial activity can be seen. The QRS complexes are very abnormal and widened to 0.20 second.

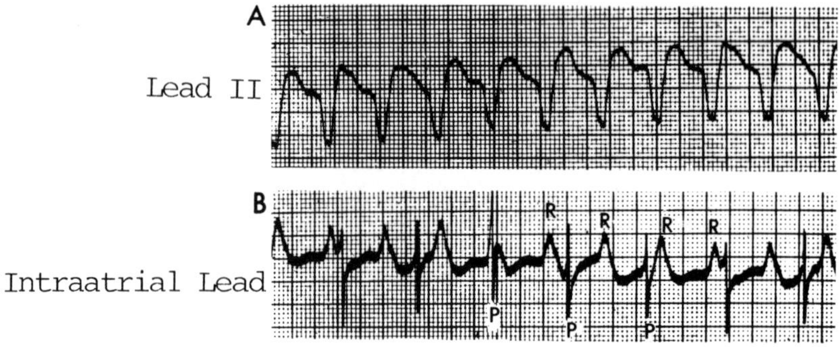

FIG 10–19.
Ventricular tachycardia. **A,** lead II demonstrates a wide QRS complex tachycardia, rate 135 beats/min, which could be either ventricular tachycardia or supraventricular tachycardia with aberration, accessory pathway, or bundle branch block. **B,** same patient showing the atrial *(P)* and ventricular *(R)* activity recorded by an intracardiac catheter in the right atrium. The atrial rate is 90 beats/min and is independent of the ventricular rate of 135 beats/min. This confirms ventricular tachycardia, which is one type of AV dissociation.

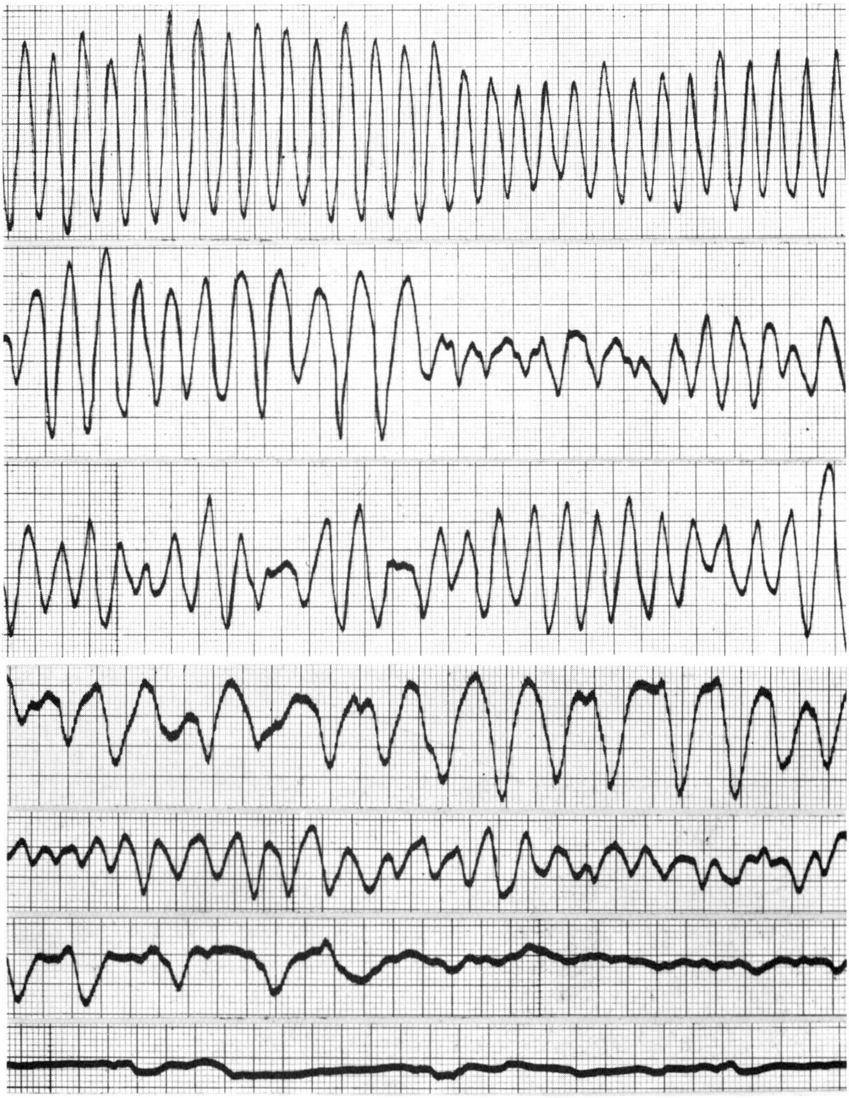

FIG 10–20.
Dying heart. Continuous strip of lead II. The *top strip* is ventricular flutter. In the *second strip,* ventricular flutter degenerates into ventricular fibrillation. In the *subsequent strips,* ventricular fibrillation merges into ventricular asystole ("straight line") and death.

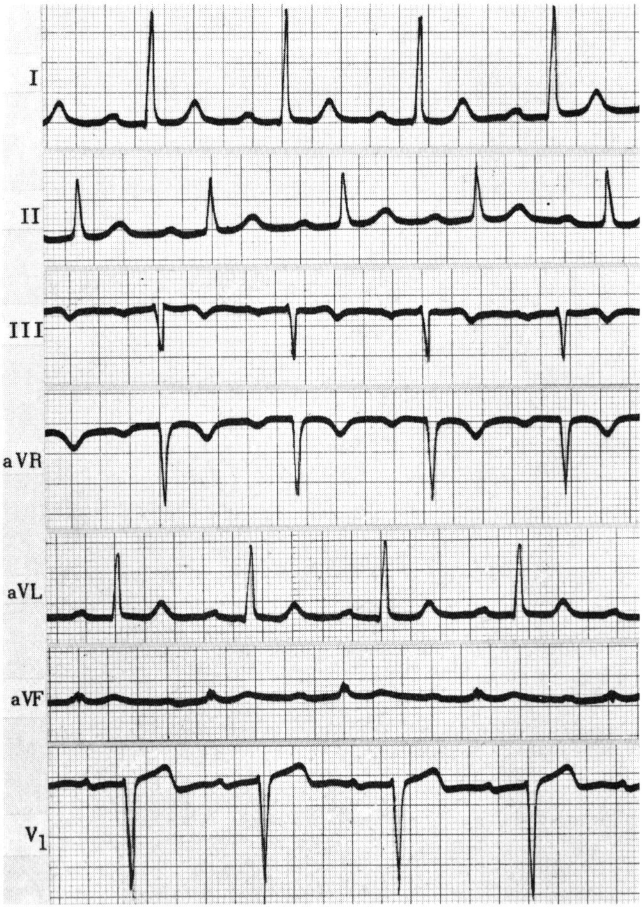

FIG 10–21.
First degree AV Block. The P-R interval is prolonged (0.28 sec). The upper limits of P-R interval in adults is considered to be 0.20 sec.

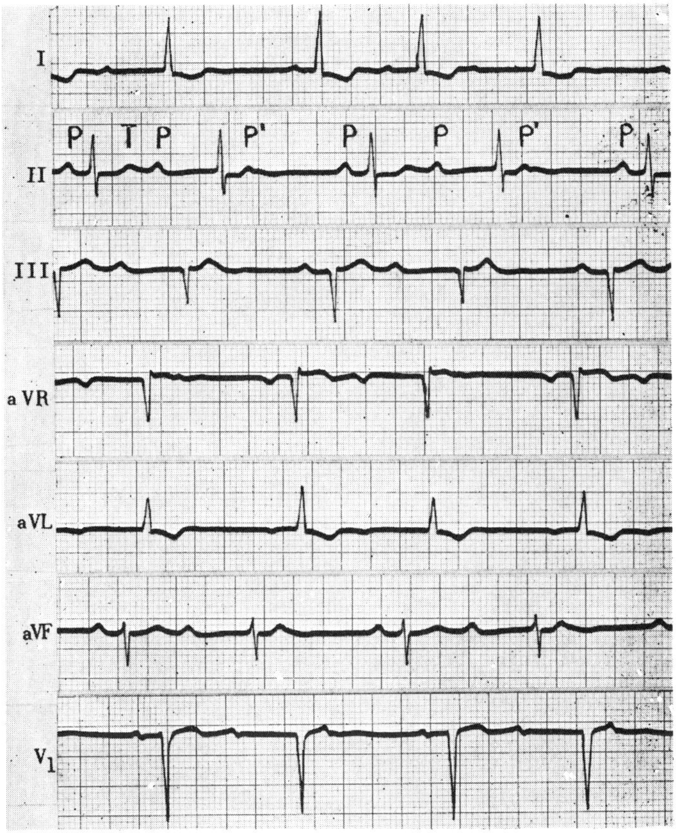

FIG 10–22.
Mobitz I (Wenckebach) second-degree AV block. Note in lead *II,* the P-P interval is constant. The P-R interval progressively increases until a blocked atrial beat (p′) occurs. This produces the grouped beating in this rhythm. The shortest P-R interval occurs after each blocked beat.

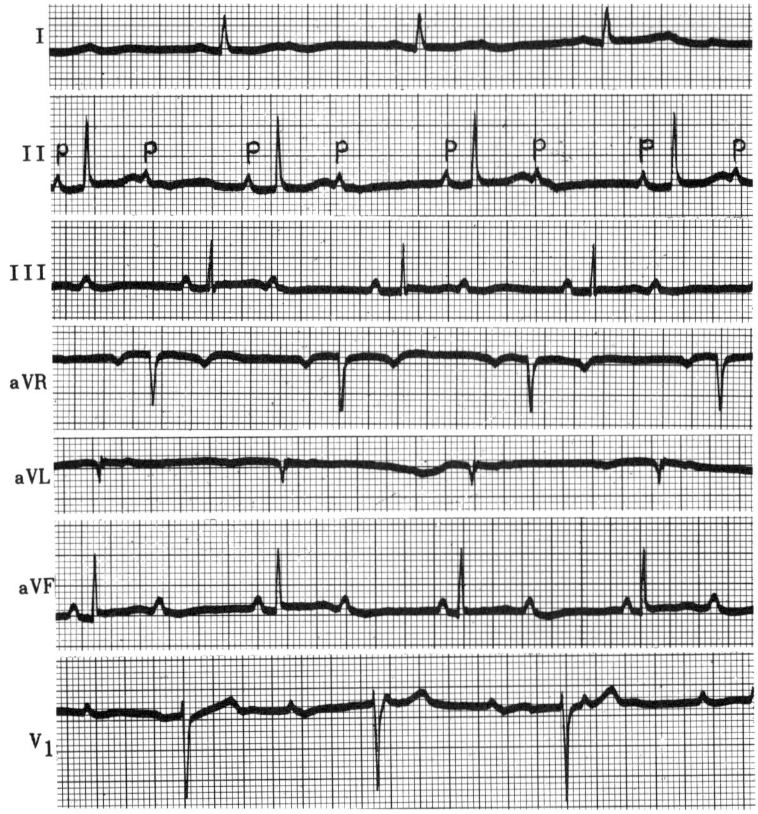

FIG 10–23.
Mobitz II second-degree AV block in leads *I* through *aVR,* then AV dissociation in leads *aVL* through V_1. In lead *II,* the atrial rate is 90 beats/min, and the ventricular rate is 45 beats/min, representing 2:1 AV block. Note the P-R intervals remain constant in the conducted atrial beats. In lead *aVF,* the P-R intervals begin to vary as the ventricular rate increases slightly to 48 beats/min. This is a type of AV dissociation when a junctional pacemaker takes over and fires independently of the atrial rate (see lead V_1). Also note in lead *II* that the P-P intervals that bound a QRS complex are slightly shorter than the P-P intervals that do not bound a QRS complex. This represents ventriculophasic sinus arrhythmia (see reference text).

CONTINUOUS MONITOR STRIP

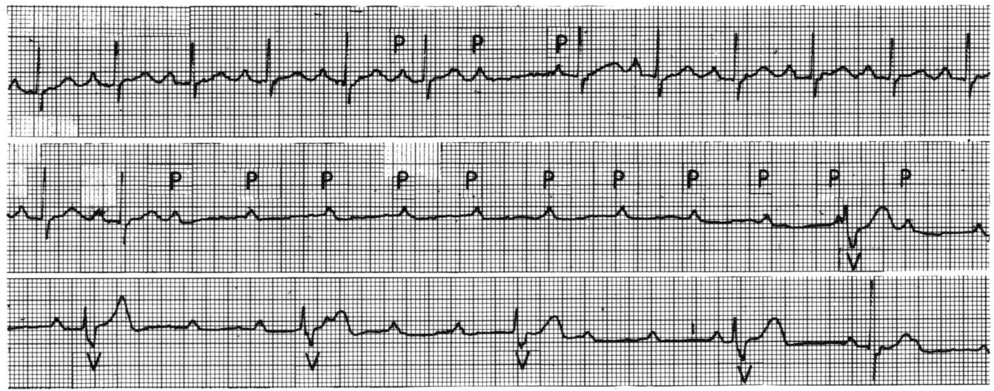

FIG 10–24.
70-year-old woman with a history of syncope. Mobitz II second-degree AV block, then complete AV block. Continuous strips from a Holter monitor. *Top strip* reveals sinus rhythm, rate 88 beats/min, and one episode of Mobitz II second-degree AV block with a blocked *P* wave and no change in the P-R intervals in the preceding or succeeding beats. The second strip reveals an episode of high-degree Mobitz II AV block that results in ventricular asystole lasting 6.2 seconds. The *bottom strip* reveals complete AV block with the atrial rate 88 beats/min and ventricular *(V)* escape rate 31 beats/min. A permanent pacemaker was inserted.

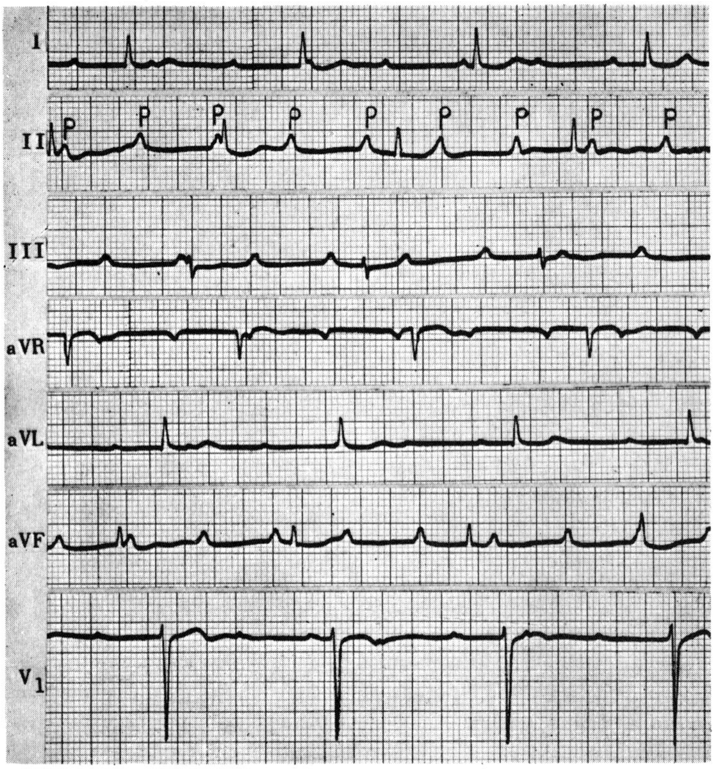

FIG 10–25.
Complete AV block. The atrial *(P)* rate is 115 beats/min, and the ventricular rate is 52 beats/min. The QRS complexes are of normal duration (less than 0.10 second), indicating that the ventricular pacemaker is located in the AV junction or bundle of His with subsequent normal ventricular conduction.

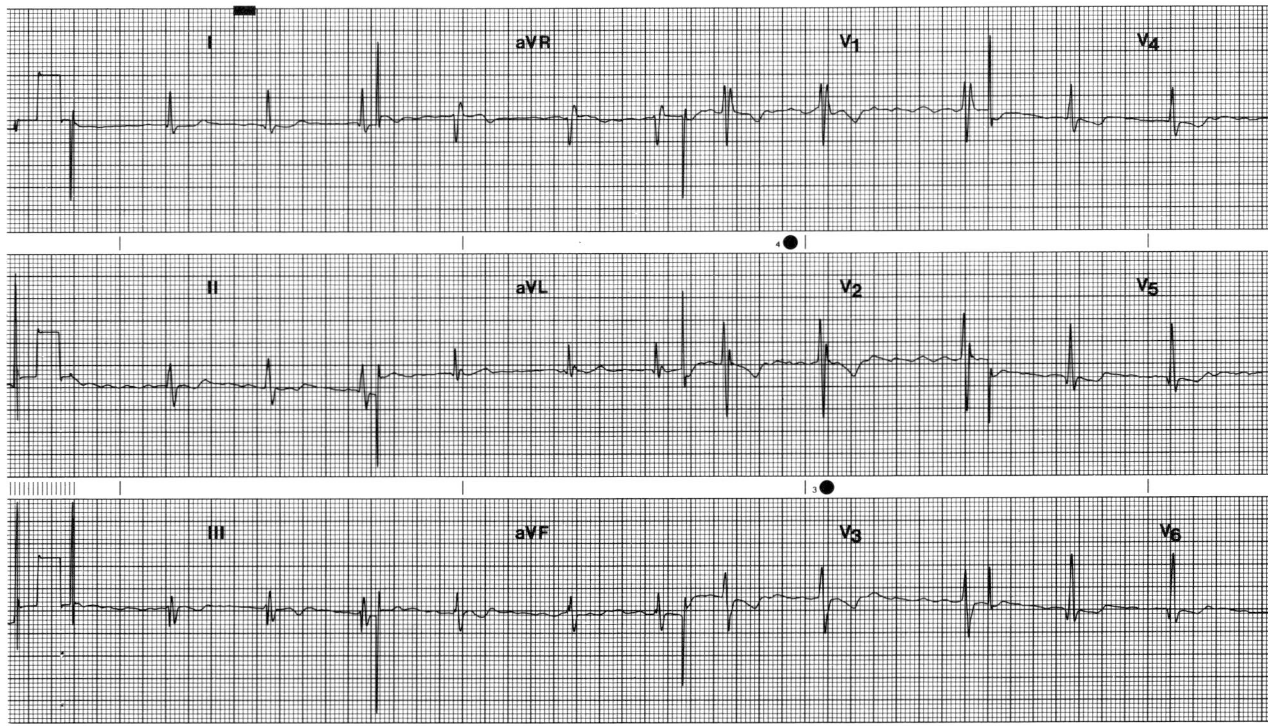

FIG 10–26.
Atrial fibrillation with incomplete right bundle branch block. 43-year-old woman taking digoxin. The rhythm is atrial fibrillation with a ventricular rate of about 70 beats/min. Note the undulating baseline, absent P waves, and irregularly irregular ventricular rate seen with atrial fibrillation. Also note the slightly prolonged QRS interval (0.11 second), the RSR′ in leads V_1 and V_2, and S waves in leads *I*, *aVL*, V_6, and repolarization changes in leads V_1 to V_3, which confirm the diagnosis of incomplete RBBB. The inferior and lateral ST-T changes reflect "Dig. effect."

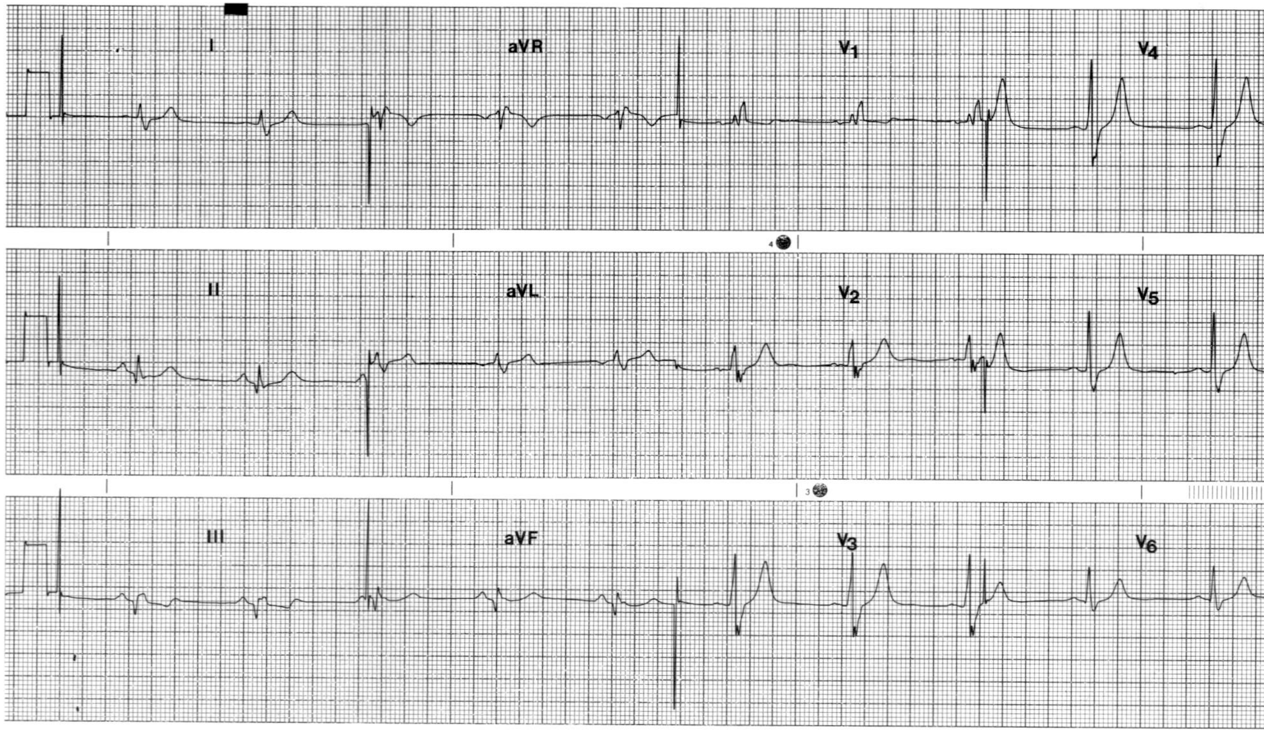

FIG 10–27.
Inferior myocardial infarction and right bundle branch block (RBBB). 69-year-old man with angina and a history of a previous myocardial infarction. Sinus rhythm, 58 beats/min. Note the Q waves in the inferior leads *(II, III, aVF)* reflecting an old inferior myocardial infarction. Also note the widened QRS complex (0.12 second), the rsR′ in V_1, the S waves in *I, aVL,* and V_6, which confirm RBBB.

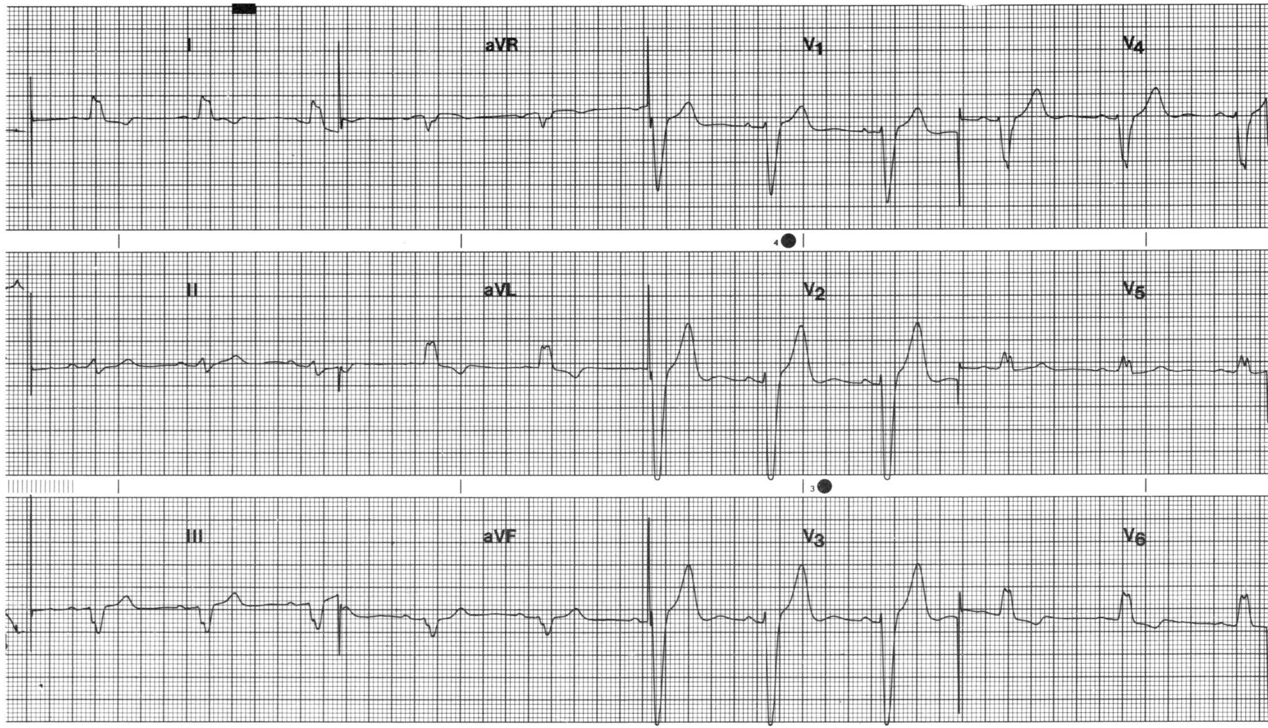

FIG 10–28.
Complete left bundle branch block (LBBB) and left axis deviation (LAD). 65-year-old woman with hypertension and renal insufficiency. Sinus rhythm, rate 60 beats/min. Note the widened QRS complex (0.14 second), the RSR′ in *I*, *aVL*, V_5, V_6 with repolarization changes and absent q waves in these same leads indicating LBBB. The small r waves in leads V_1 through V_4 are consistent with LBBB and should not be confused with an old anterior myocardial infarction. LAD (QRS axis −40°).

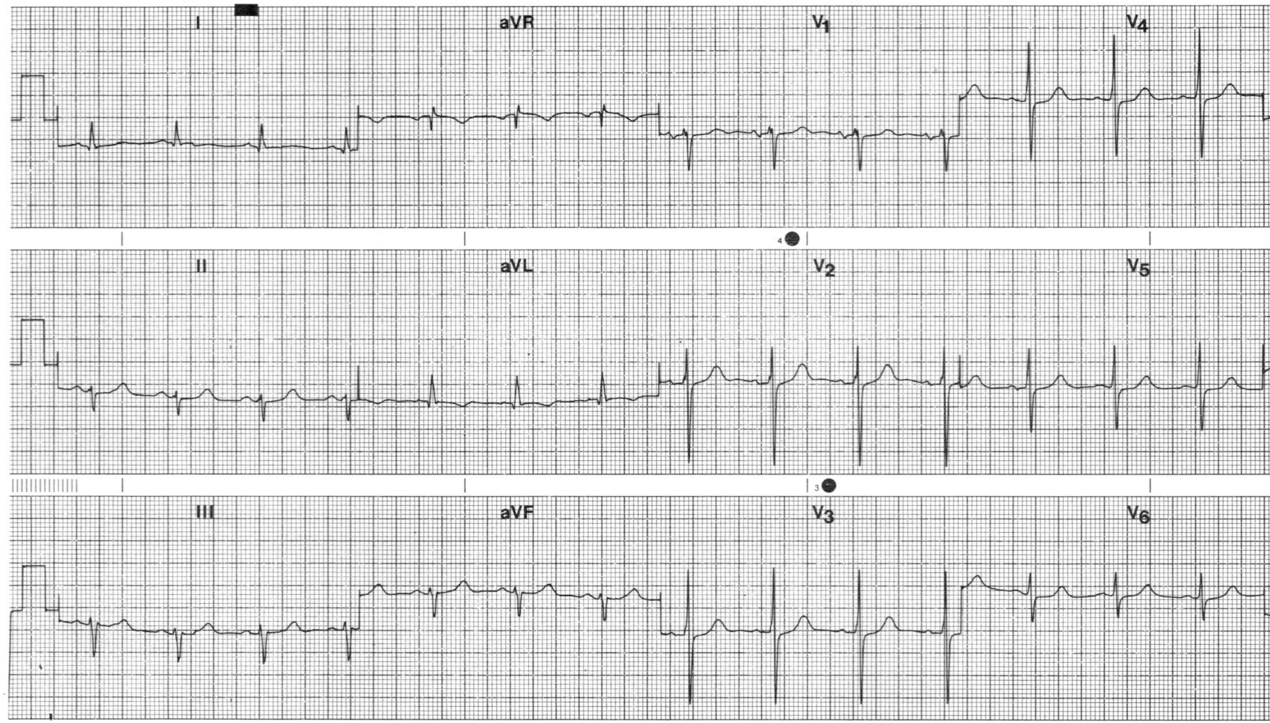

FIG 10–29.
Left anterior fascicular block (LAFB). 77-year-old man with no prior clinical history of heart disease. Sinus rhythm, rate 82 beats/min. Note the small q and large R waves in *I* and *aVL,* the small r and deep S waves in *II, III,* and *aVF,* and the left axis deviation (LAD) of −50° consistent with the diagnosis of LAFB.

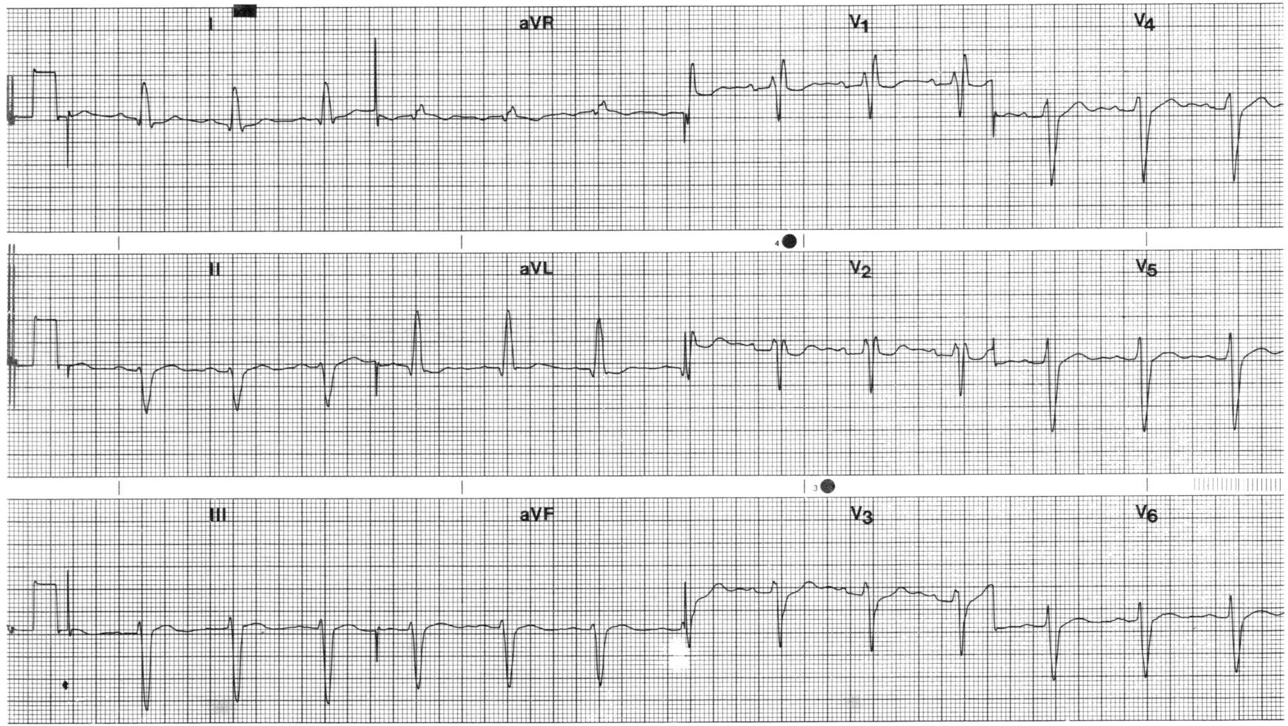

FIG 10–30.

Right bundle branch block and left anterior fascicular block (bifascicular block). 75-year-old man with hypertension, angina, and congestive heart failure. Sinus rhythm, rate 75 beats/min; first-degree AV block (P-R 0.22 second). Note the wide QRS (0.12 second), rsR′ in V_1 and V_2, and the deep S waves in *I* and V_6 indicating RBBB. Also note the QRS axis (−75°), the small q and large R waves in *I* and *aVL*, and the small r and deep S waves in *II*, *III*, *aVF*, indicating LAFB. The combination of RBBB and LAFB is called *bifascicular block*.

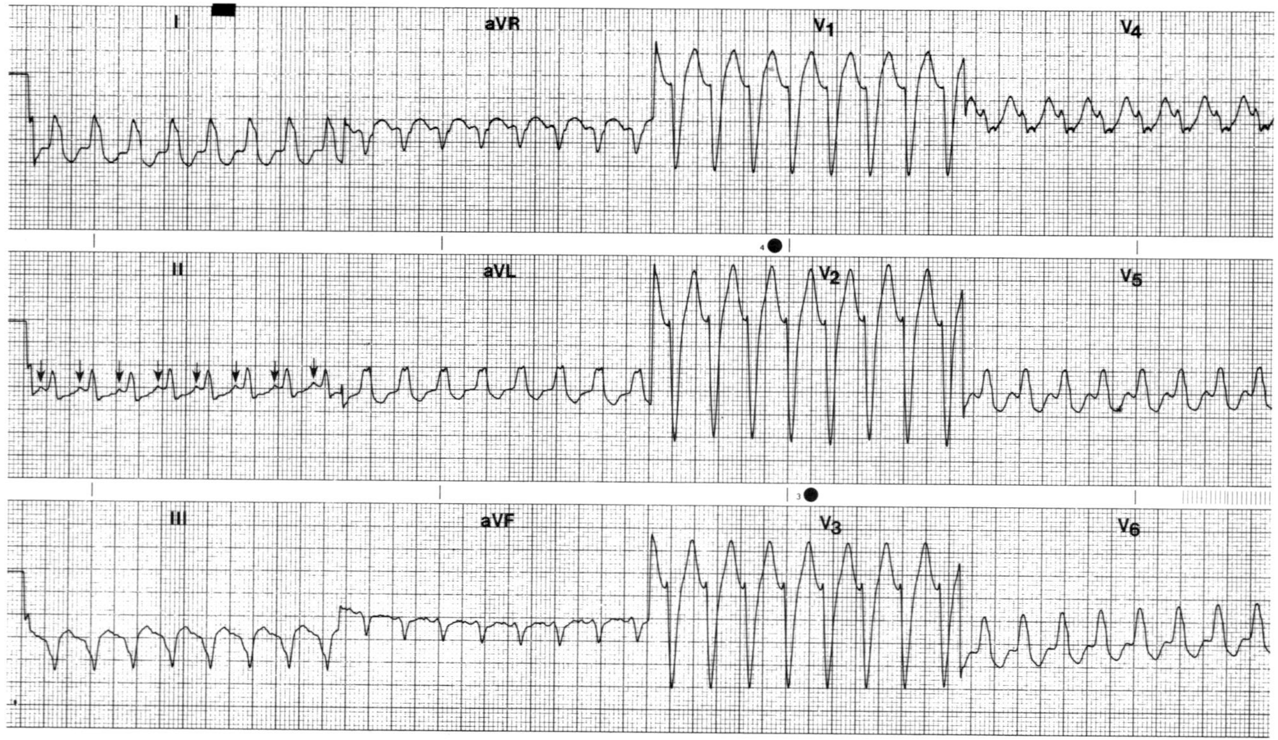

FIG 10–31.
Wide QRS tachycardia. 73-year-old man who had a normal ECG before knee operation. Postoperatively, he was found to be hypotensive with this ECG. Wide QRS complex tachycardia, rate 180 beats/min. The possible diagnoses include ventricular tachycardia or supraventricular tachycardia with aberration, accessory pathway, or bundle branch block. The presence of atrial waves between the QRS complexes (best seen in lead *II*) is consistent with a supraventricular tachycardia (possibly sinus tachycardia, atrial flutter, or junctional reentrant tachycardia). The wide QRS complexes may be secondary to aberration or an accessory pathway; however, a rate-dependent LBBB is more likely. When sinus rhythm was restored the following day, the QRS width returned to its previously normal duration.

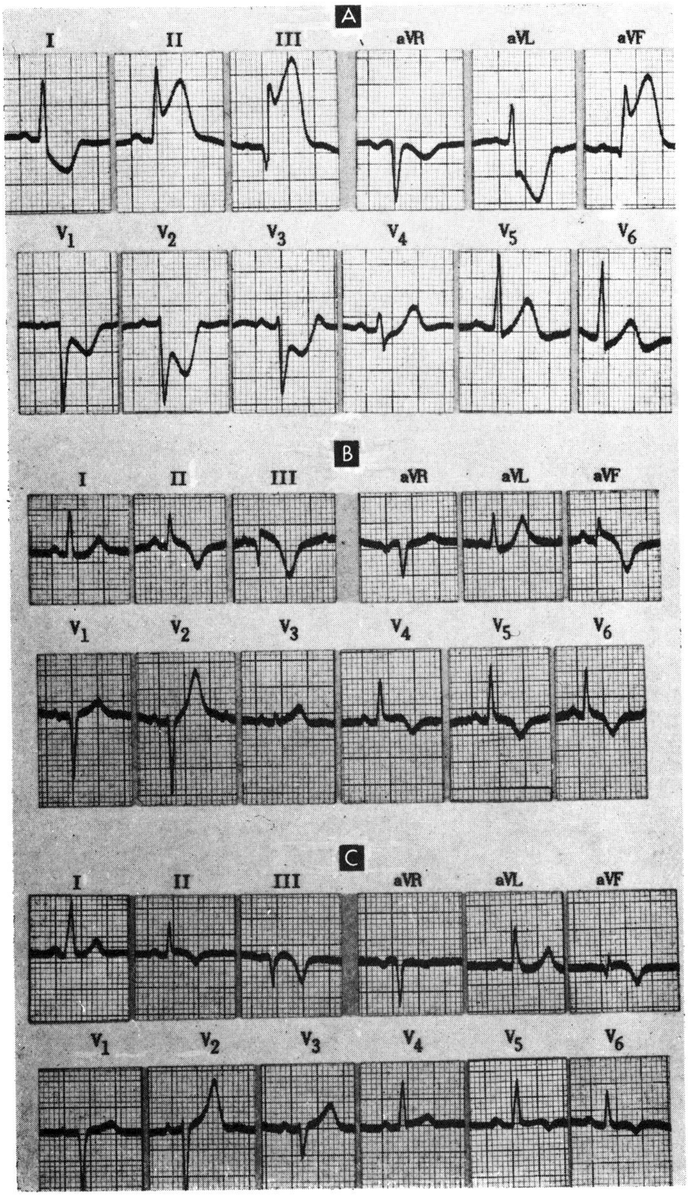

FIG 10–32.
Acute inferior myocardial infarction. **A,** 3 hours after the onset of chest pain. Note the elevated ST segments in the inferior leads *(II, III, aVF)* with reciprocal ST depression in leads *I, aVL,* V_1, V_2, V_3. **B,** 24 hours later. Note the less marked ST elevation but with deeply inverted T waves and the beginning of Q waves in the inferior leads. The reciprocal ST changes have resolved; however, there is new ST elevation with T wave inversion in leads V_4 to V_6 demonstrating lateral wall extension of the infarction. **C,** 5 days later, showing the evolutionary changes. The Q wave in V_1 and poor R wave progression in V_1 through V_3 in all three tracings is consistent with an old anteroseptal myocardial infarction.

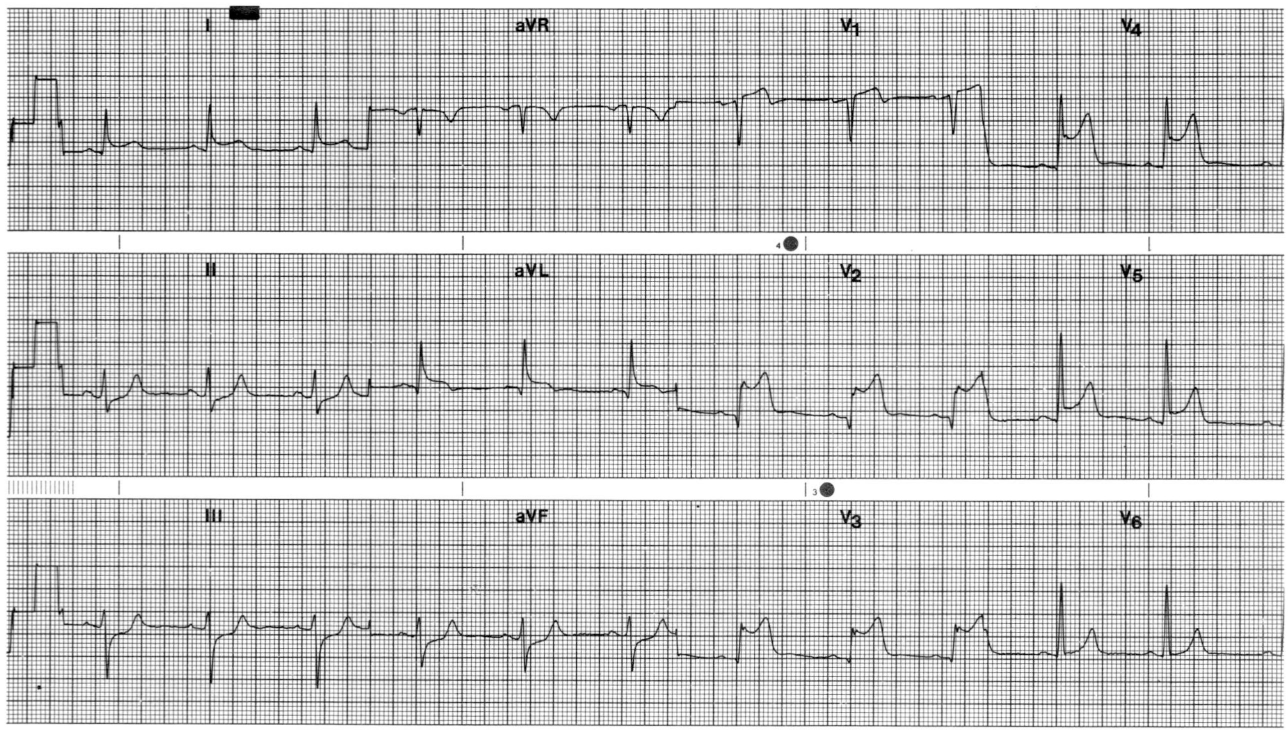

FIG 10–33.
Acute anterior myocardial infarction. 46-year-old man with 2 hours of chest pain. Note the ST elevation in leads V_1 through V_6 and *I, aVL* with the beginning of Q waves in leads V_1 through V_4 demonstrating acute anterior myocardial infarction. Also note the reciprocal ST depression in the inferior leads *(II, III, aVF)*. Cardiac catheterization revealed total occlusion of the proximal anterior descending coronary artery.

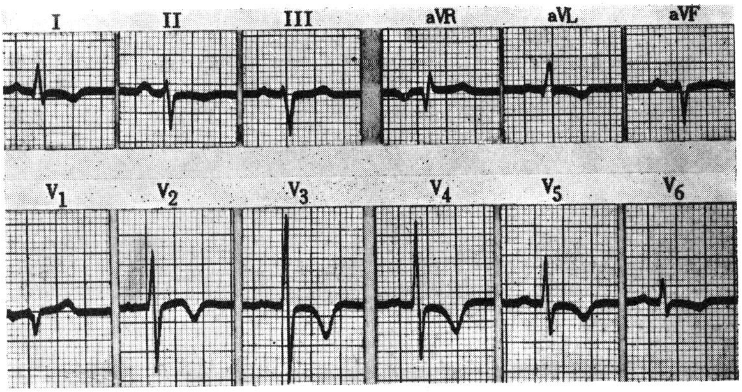

FIG 10–34.
Acute anterolateral subendocardial (non Q wave) infarction and left anterior fascicular block (LAFB). Note the ST depression and symmetrical T wave inversion in leads V_2 through V_6 and *I, aVL* without ST elevation. Additionally, the absence of Q waves and the clinical setting of chest pain and elevated cardiac enzymes are consistent with the diagnosis of subendocardial (non Q wave) myocardial infarction. The marked LAD (QRS axis −60°), small q and tall R waves in *I* and *aVL,* and small r and deep S waves in *II, III, aVF* indicate LAFB.

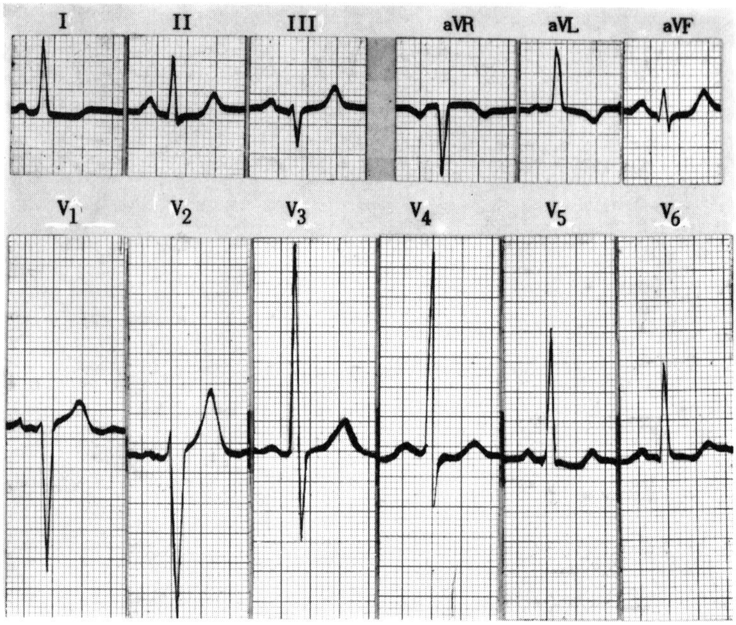

FIG 10–35.
Left ventricular hypertrophy (LVH). 49-year-old man with a blood pressure of 260/115 mm Hg. Note the increased QRS voltage (deep S in V_1, tall R in V_5); depressed ST and inverted T waves in *I, aVL,* V_5, V_6; and widened QRS complex (0.10 second). QRS axis is +15°.

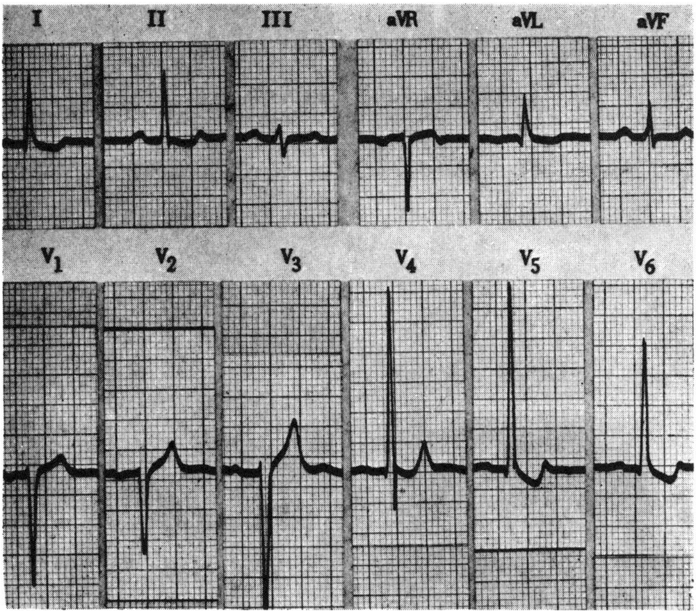

FIG 10–36.
Left ventricular hypertrophy (LVH). "Dig. effect." Observe the increased QRS voltage (deep S in V_1, tall R in V_5), and the ST-T changes in leads V_5 and V_6. The patient was taking digoxin, which resulted in the "scooped" ST depression in the lateral leads. QRS axis is +30°.

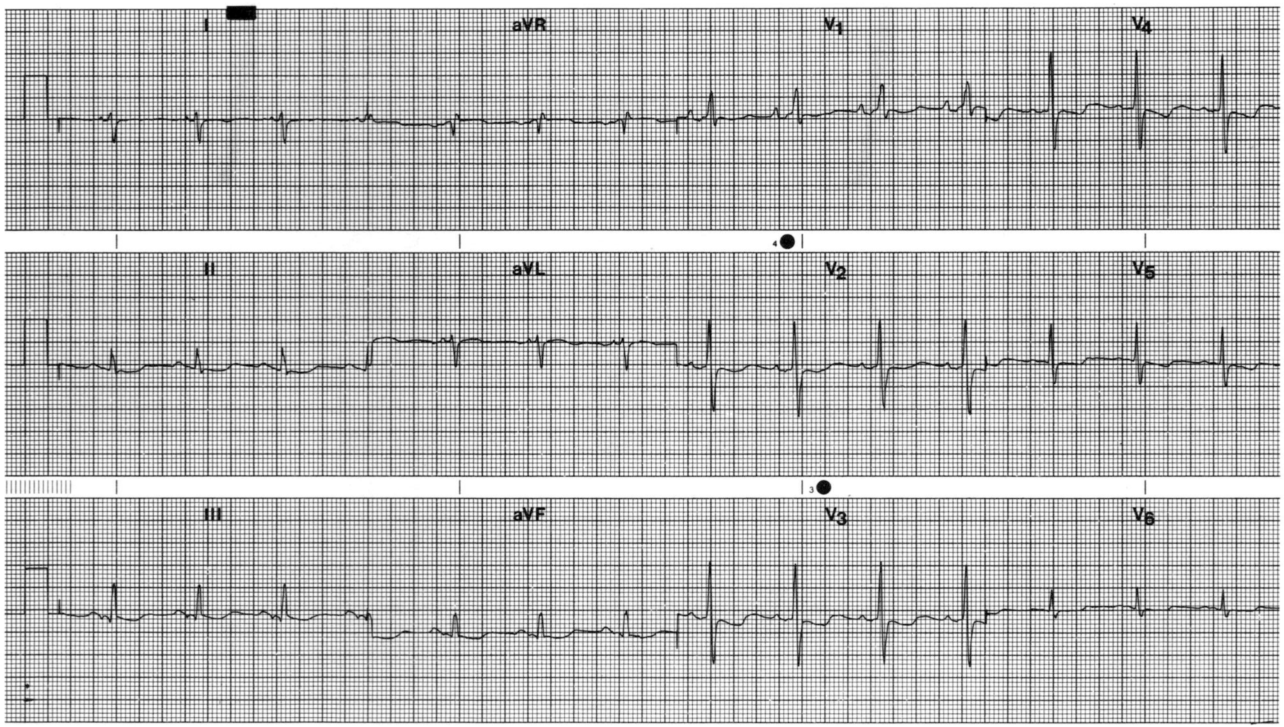

FIG 10–37.
Right ventricular hypertrophy (RVH). 49-year-old man with mitral stenosis. Sinus rhythm, rate 82 beats/min, left atrial hypertrophy. The broad, notched P waves in the inferior leads *(II, III, aVF)* suggest left atrial hypertrophy. Note the right axis deviation (QRS axis +110°) and the R:S ratio in lead V_1 greater than one, which are consistent with RVH. The diffuse ST-T changes are secondary to "Dig. effect."

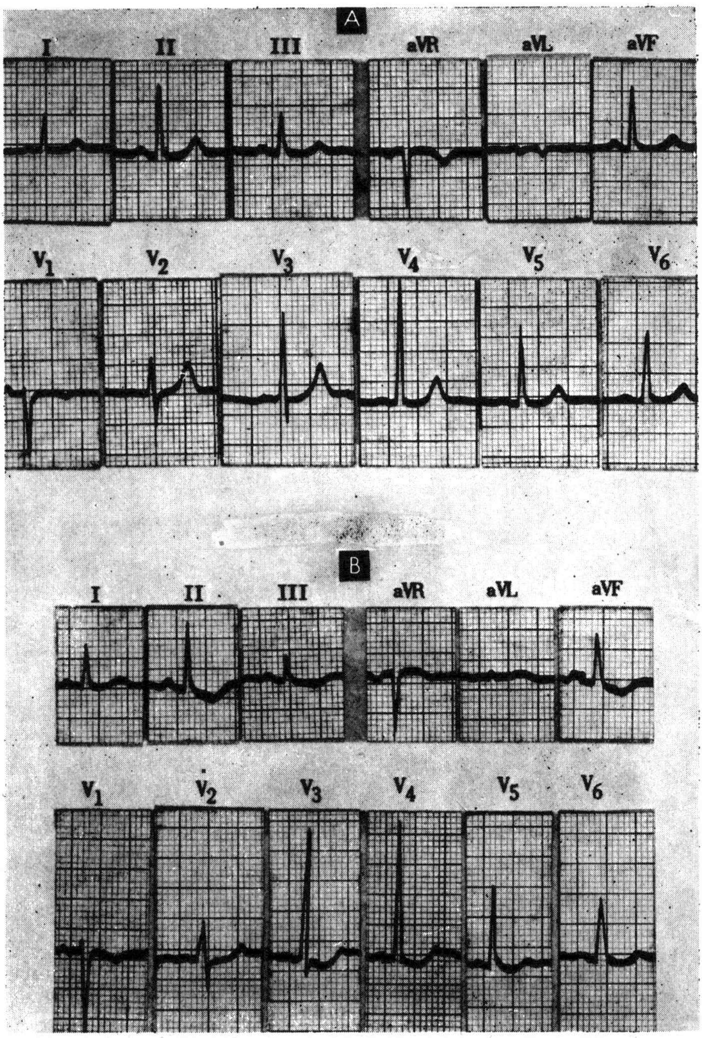

FIG 10–38.
"Dig. effect." **A,** before digoxin. **B,** after digoxin, showing typical ST and T wave changes. Also note the slight P-R interval lengthening and the slight Q-T interval shortening consistent with "Dig. effect."

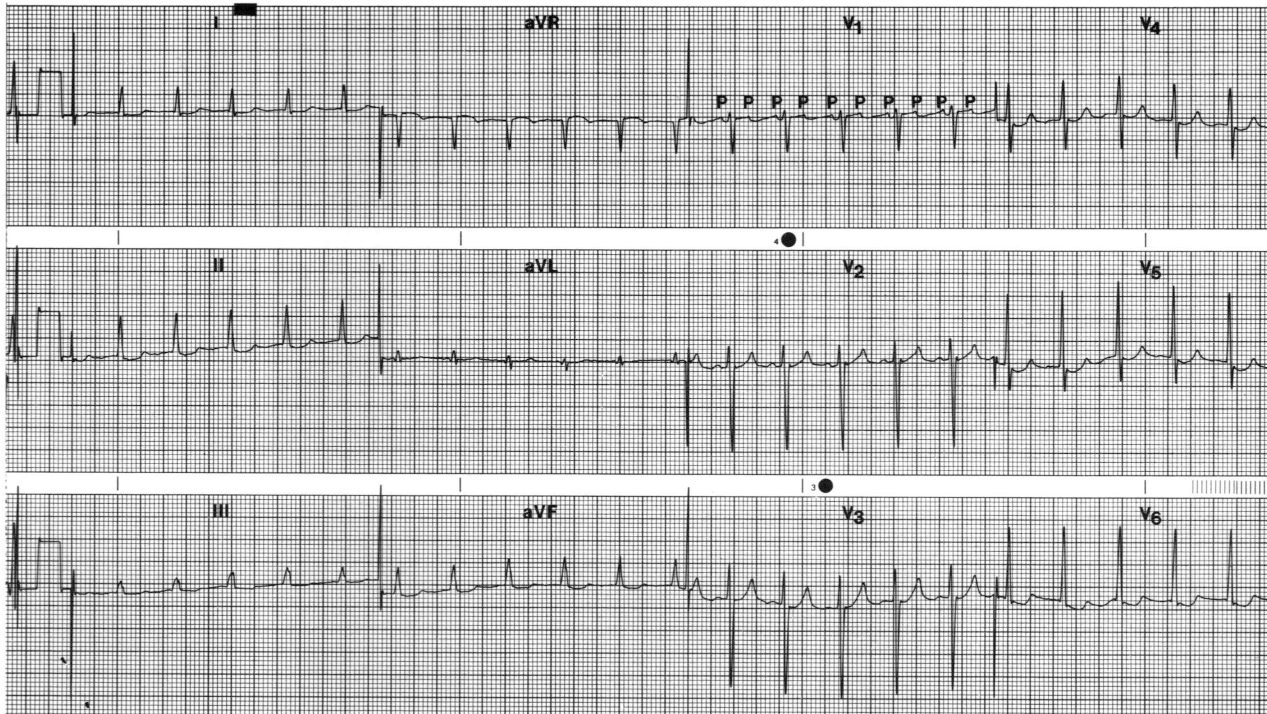

FIG 10–39.
Supraventricular tachycardia (SVT); atrial tachycardia with 2:1 AV block. 62-year-old woman taking digoxin, who had rheumatic heart disease, mitral valve replacement, congestive heart failure, and atrial fibrillation. She developed "Dig. toxicity" resulting in atrial tachycardia with 2:1 AV block. The P waves are difficult to identify, but close inspection of lead V_1 reveals regular P wave deflections *(P)* at a rate of 250 beats/min. The ventricular rate is 125 beats/min. Another possible diagnosis would be sinus tachycardia if the P waves superimposed on the T waves in lead V_1 had not been seen. Note the sagging ST segments in the inferior and lateral leads secondary to "Dig effect."

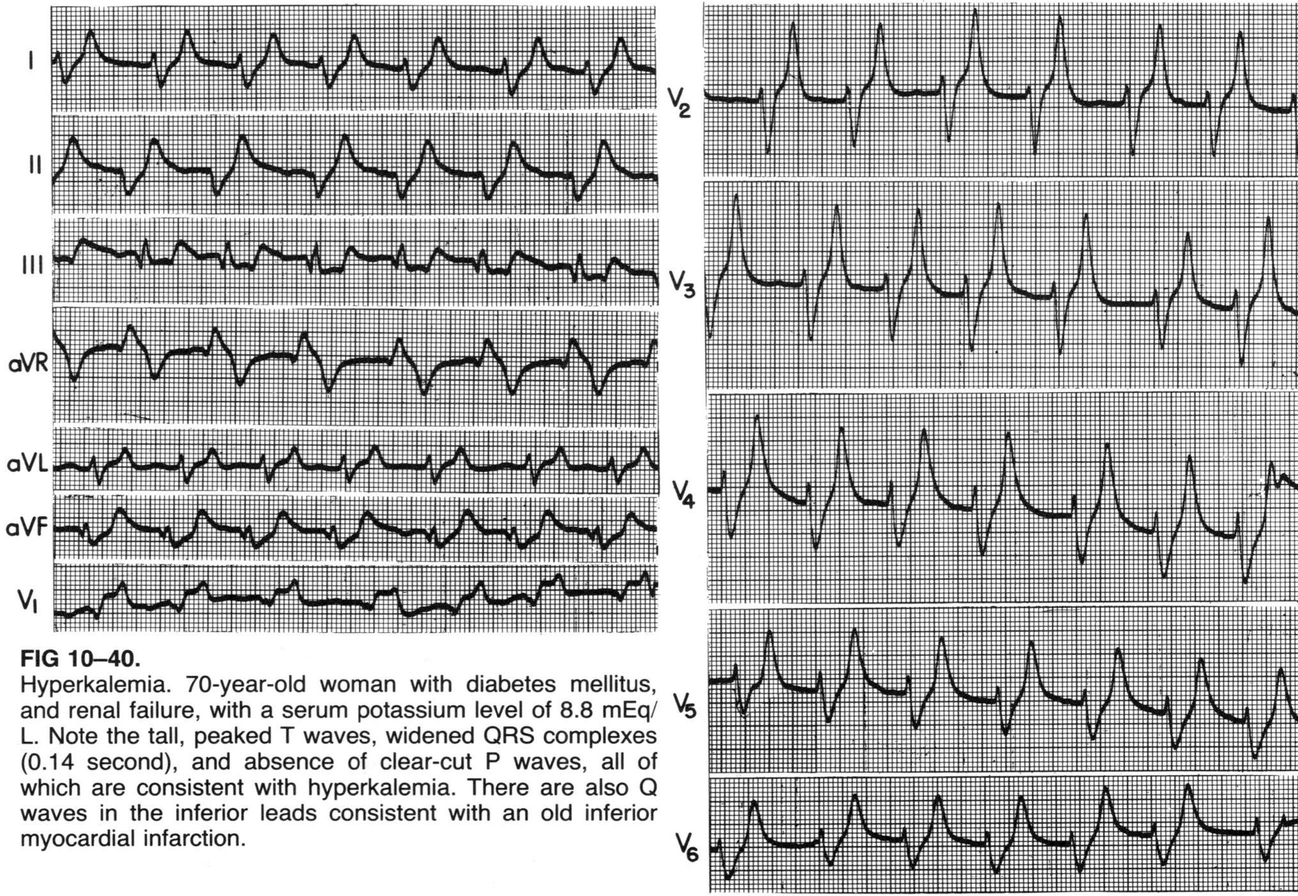

FIG 10–40.
Hyperkalemia. 70-year-old woman with diabetes mellitus, and renal failure, with a serum potassium level of 8.8 mEq/L. Note the tall, peaked T waves, widened QRS complexes (0.14 second), and absence of clear-cut P waves, all of which are consistent with hyperkalemia. There are also Q waves in the inferior leads consistent with an old inferior myocardial infarction.

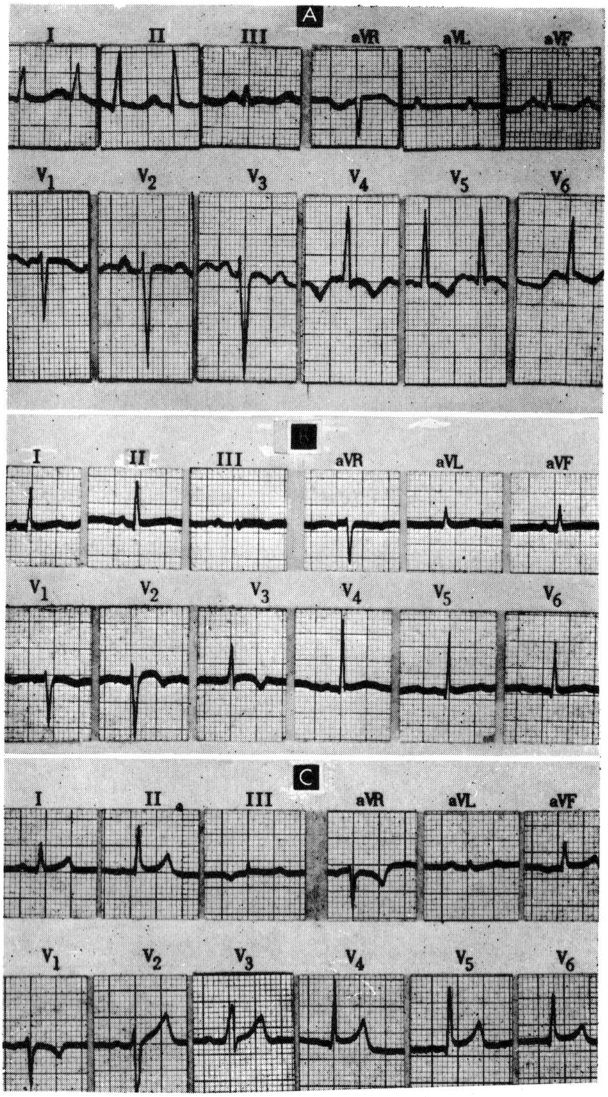

FIG 10–41.
Hypokalemia. 17-year-old woman with diabetic ketoacidosis and serum potassium level of 2.2 mEq/L. **A,** the immediate period of hypokalemia demonstrating depressed ST segments, inverted T waves, and prominent U waves in almost all the leads, especially V_2 through V_5. **B,** 2 days later after potassium replacement. The ST segments and T waves are returning to normal. **C,** 5 days after treatment demonstrating baseline ST segments and upright T waves with a normal potassium level of 4.5 mEq/L. Note early repolarization in leads *I, II,* V_4 to V_6, which is a normal variant.

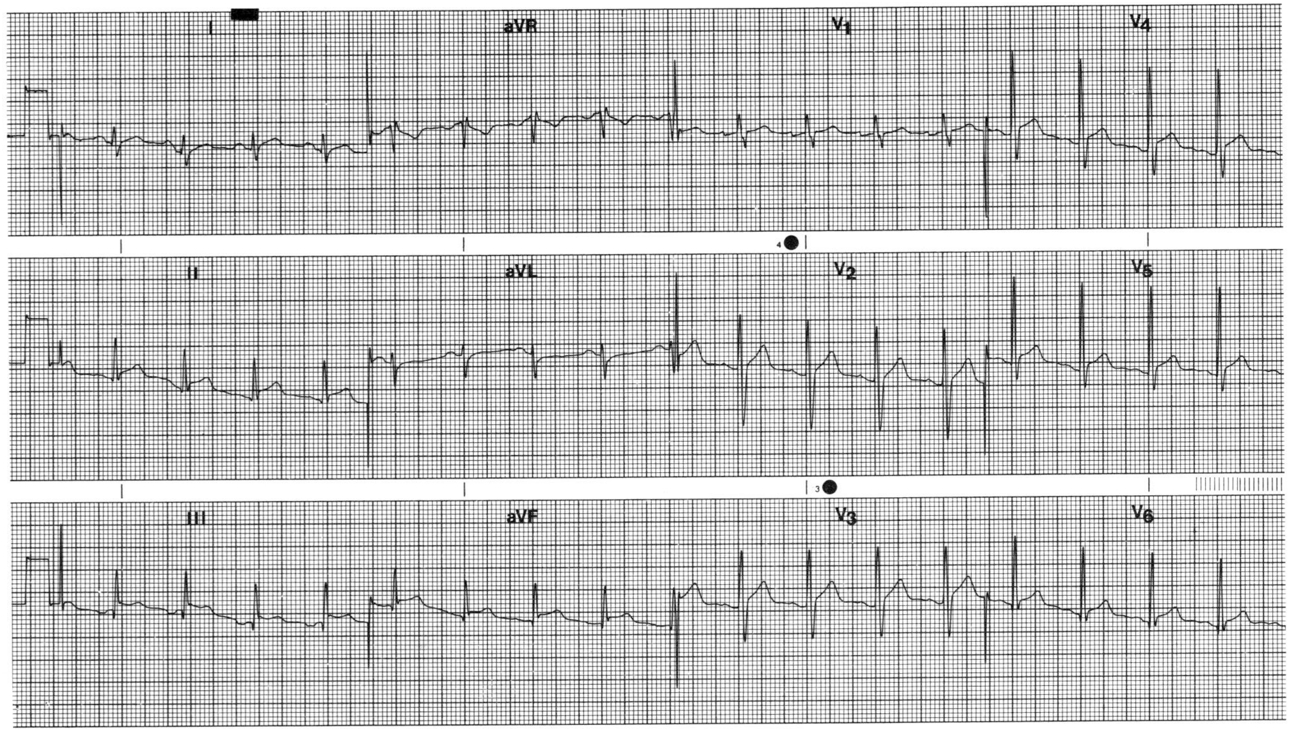

FIG 10–42.
Acute pericarditis. 21-year-old man with sharp, stabbing chest pain for 2 days and a pericardial friction rub on admission. Observe the ST elevation in every lead except *aVR*, supporting the diagnosis of acute pericarditis. This ECG should not be confused with acute myocardial infarction, which does not have diffuse ST elevation. The clinical data was very helpful in this case. Serial ECGs confirmed the diagnosis of acute pericarditis.

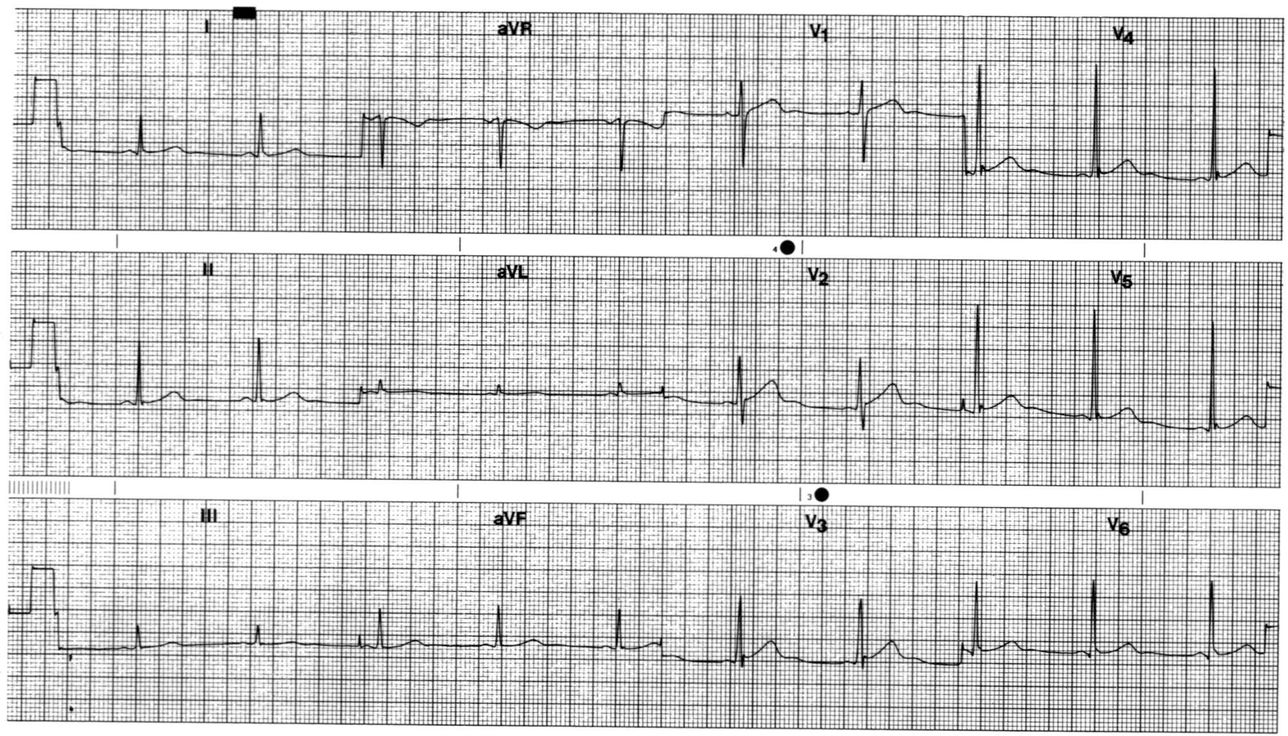

FIG 10–43.
Early repolarization, a normal ECG variant. 42-year-old man with no history of heart disease. Note the elevated ST segments with a notch in the J point in leads V_2 to V_5. The ST elevation did not change with serial tracings.

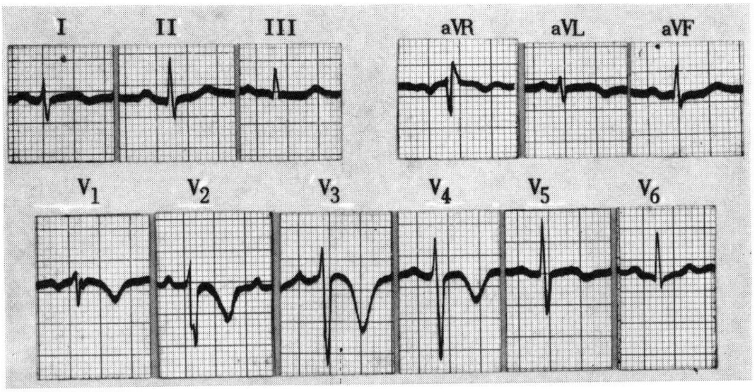

FIG 10–44.
Acute pulmonary embolism. 41-year-old patient with sudden onset of chest pain and shortness of breath 10 days after abdominal operation. The characteristic changes include deep inverted T waves V_1 to V_4 (right ventricular ischemia); RAD (+100°); rsr′ in V_1 (incomplete right bundle branch block). Early ECGs and serial ECGs are important in the diagnosis of pulmonary embolism.

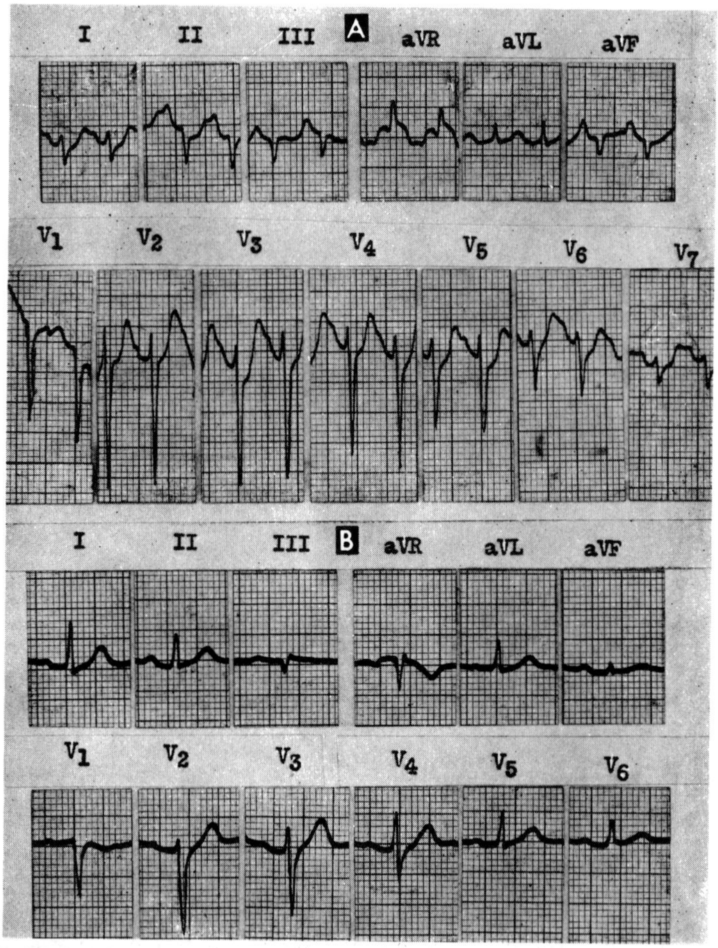

FIG 10–45.
Pulmonary embolus, acute cor pulmonale, and paroxysmal atrial tachycardia (PAT). 23-year-old woman, 3 days postpartum, with acute chest pain and shortness of breath. Pulmonary embolus with acute cor pulmonale and PAT, rate 180 beats/min. **A,** the rhythm is PAT at a rate of 180 beats/min. Note the extreme RAD (QRS axis $-105°$), the $S_1Q_3T_3$ pattern, the poor R wave progression, and the depressed ST segments V_3 to V_6, indicating anterior or right ventricular wall ischemia. The Q waves inferiorly *(II, III, aVF)*, which are suggestive of inferior infarction, in this case are consistent with pulmonary embolism. **B,** 1 day later, normal ECG. All previous acute changes have resolved.

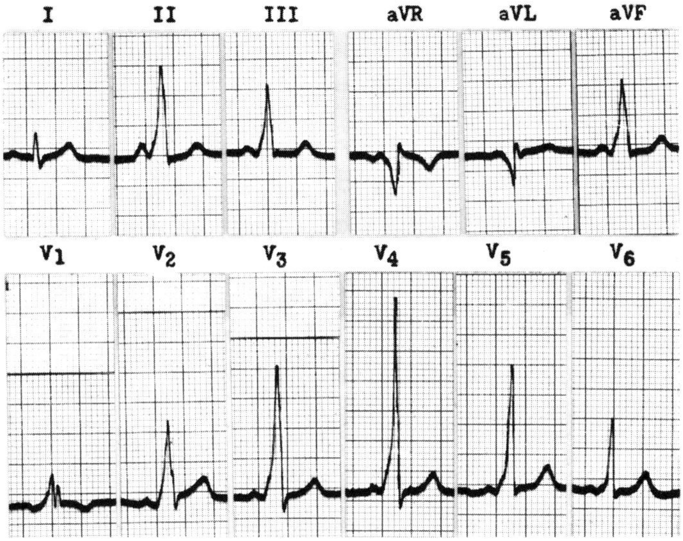

FIG 10–46.
Wolff-Parkinson-White (WPW) syndrome, type A. Note the short P-R interval (0.10 second) and the wide QRS (0.12 second) resulting from the delta wave. The predominantly positive QRS deflections in leads V_1 and V_2 indicate type A WPW syndrome.

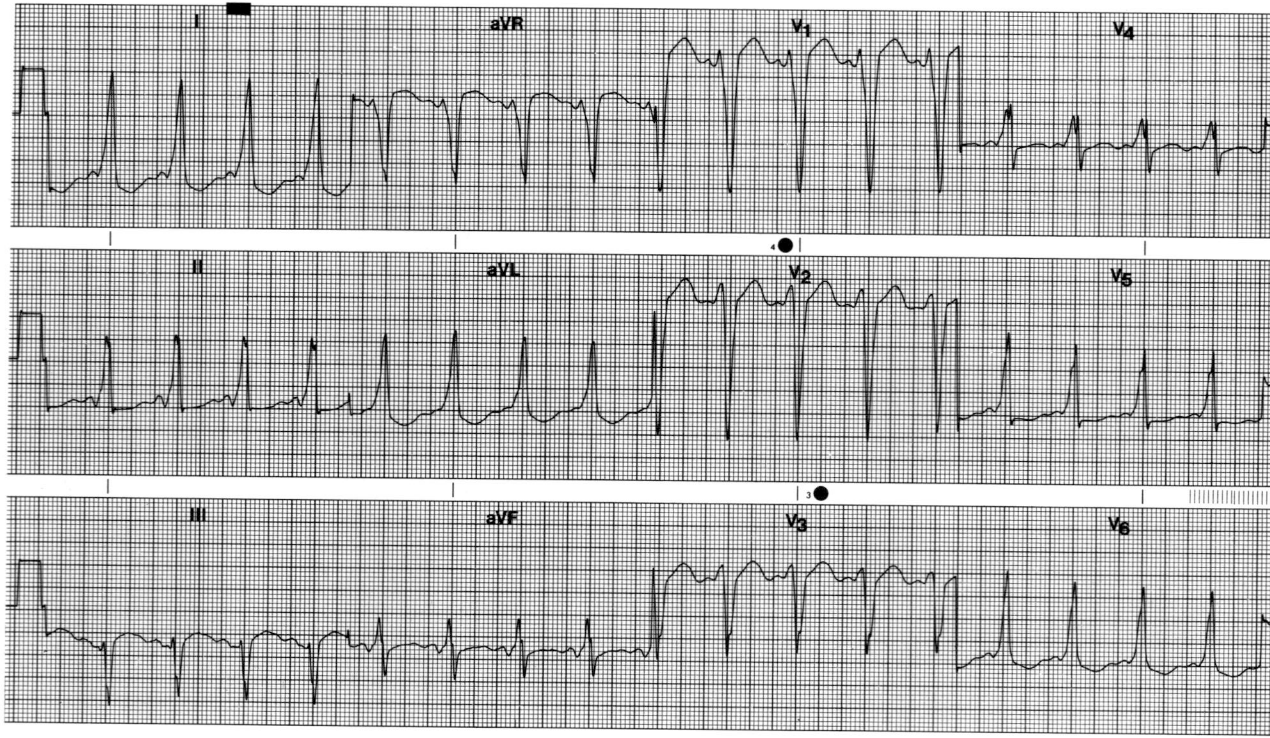

FIG 10–47.
Wolff Parkinson White (WPW) syndrome, type B. Note the short P-R interval (0.08 second), the wide QRS complex (0.16 second) because of the initial delta wave, and the abnormal repolarization changes. This could be mistaken for left ventricular hypertrophy. The predominantly negative QRS deflections in leads V_1 and V_2 indicate type B WPW syndrome.

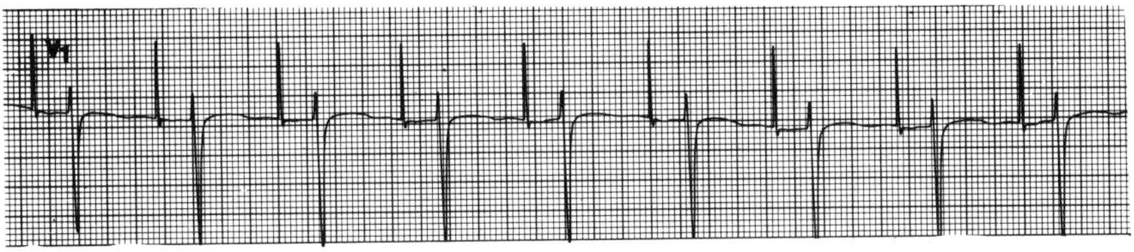

FIG 10–48.
Atrial pacemaker recorded in lead V_1. Note the atrial pacemaker spike preceding each P-QRS-T complex at a rate of 70 beats/min.

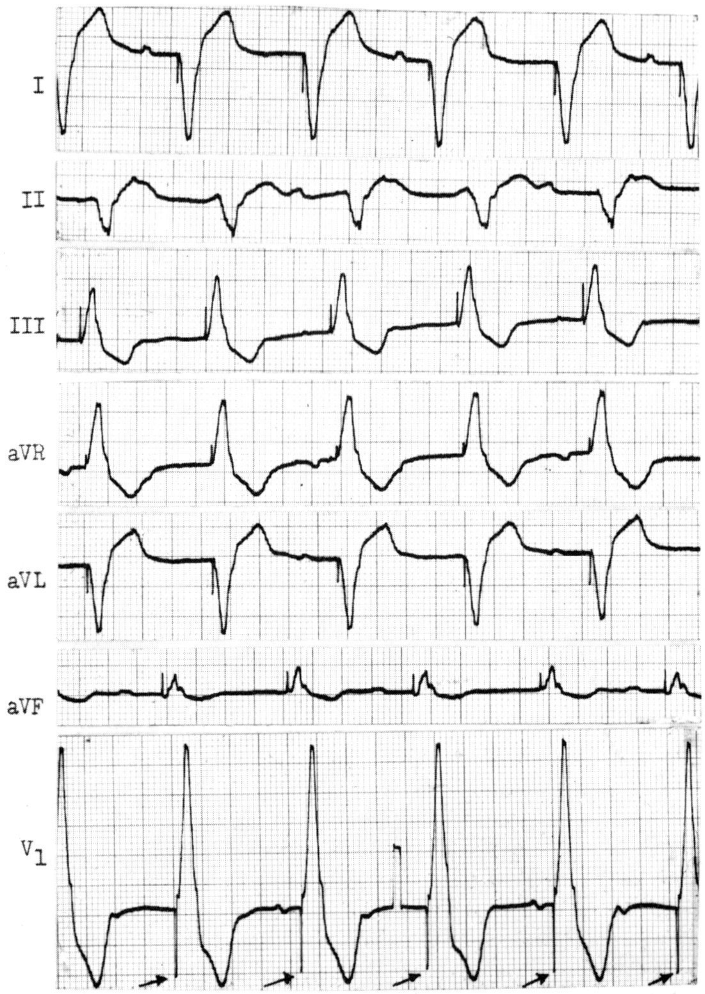

FIG 10–49.
Ventricular pacemaker, epicardially implanted. Note the ventricular pacemaker spikes (*arrows* in V_1) immediately preceding each QRS complex at a rate of 70 beats/min. The QRS morphology resembles right bundle branch block that is characteristic of a left ventricular epicardial pacemaker. There are nonconducted P waves periodically seen throughout the strips (note lead II).

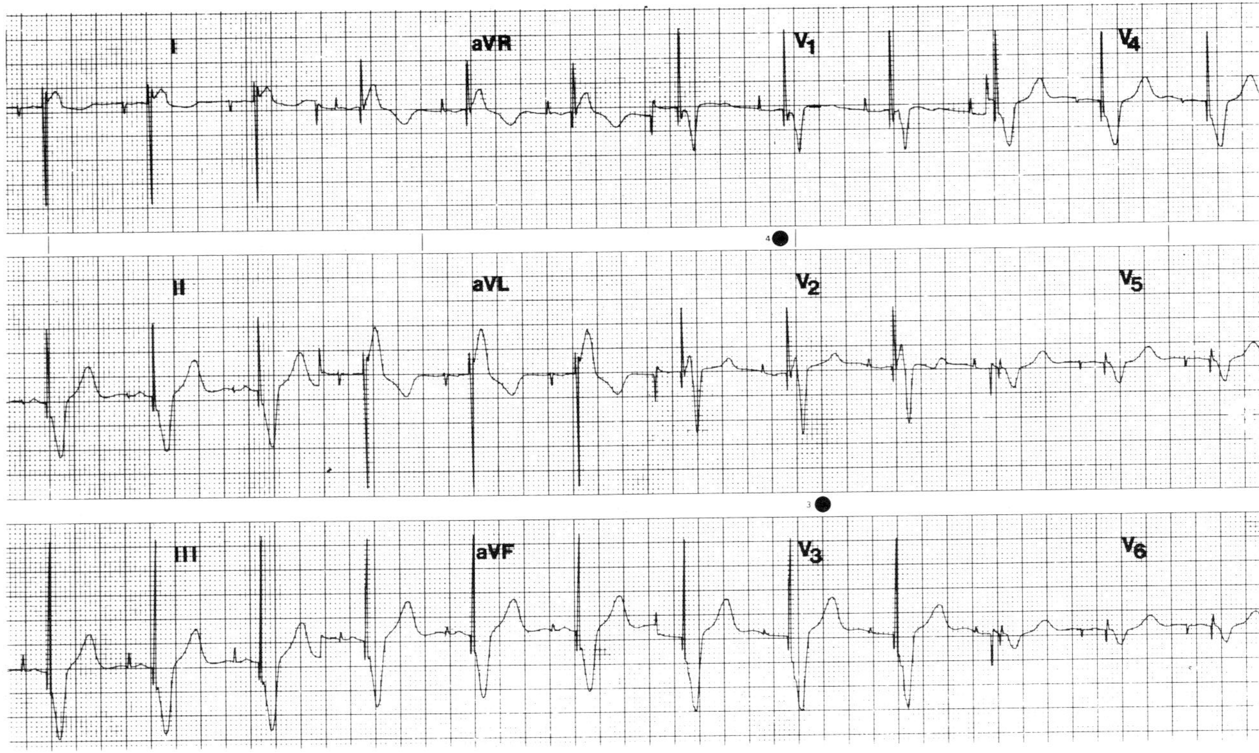

FIG 10–50.
Dual chamber, DDD, pacemaker. The leads are in the right atrium and right ventricle. Note the small atrial pacemaker spikes preceding the P waves, an AV delay of 0.20 second, and the ventricular pacemaker spikes preceding each QRS complex at a rate of 70 beats/min.

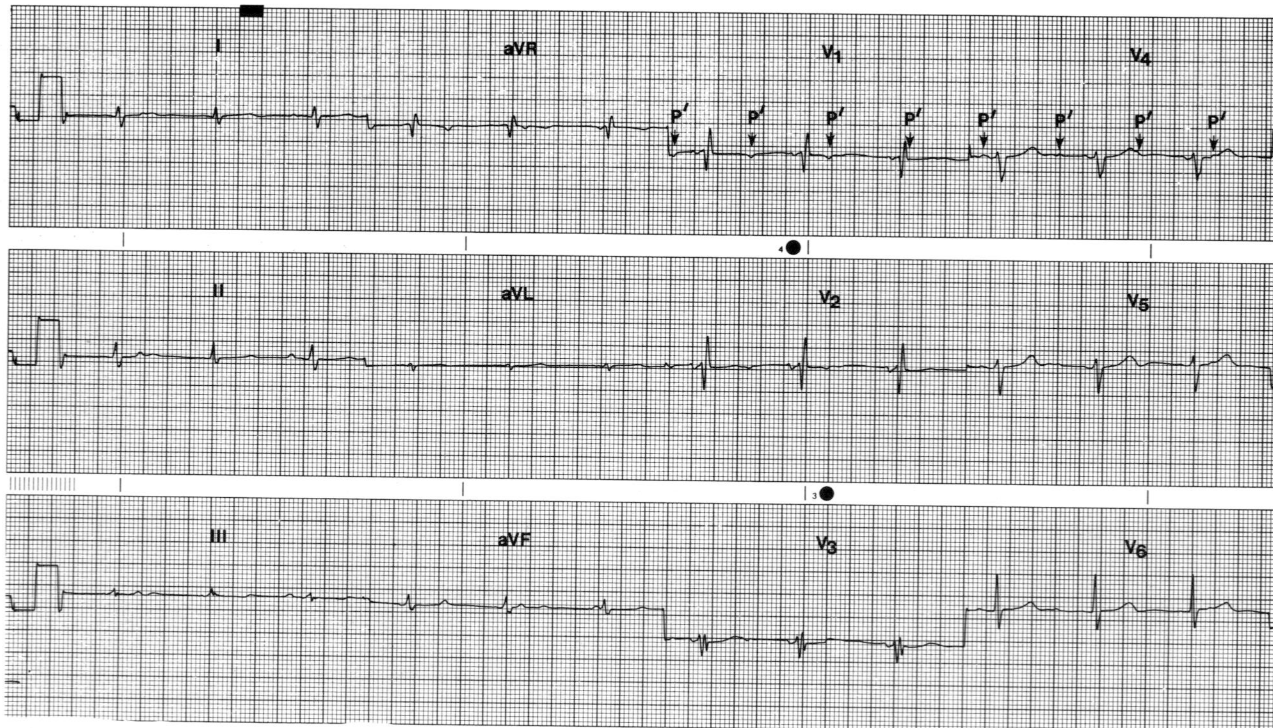

FIG 10–51.

Cardiac transplantation. 19-year-old male, 1 month after cardiac transplant. The new donor heart rhythm is sinus, rate 70 beats/min, rightward axis (QRS axis +90°), incomplete RBBB. A careful search reveals P waves *(P′)* that beat independently of the new donor rhythm. This is a parasystolic atrial rhythm, rate 85 beats/min, which comes from the remnant SA node remaining in the part of the right atrium that is connected to the new donor heart. This rhythm is often seen after cardiac transplantation and usually extinguishes itself in time.

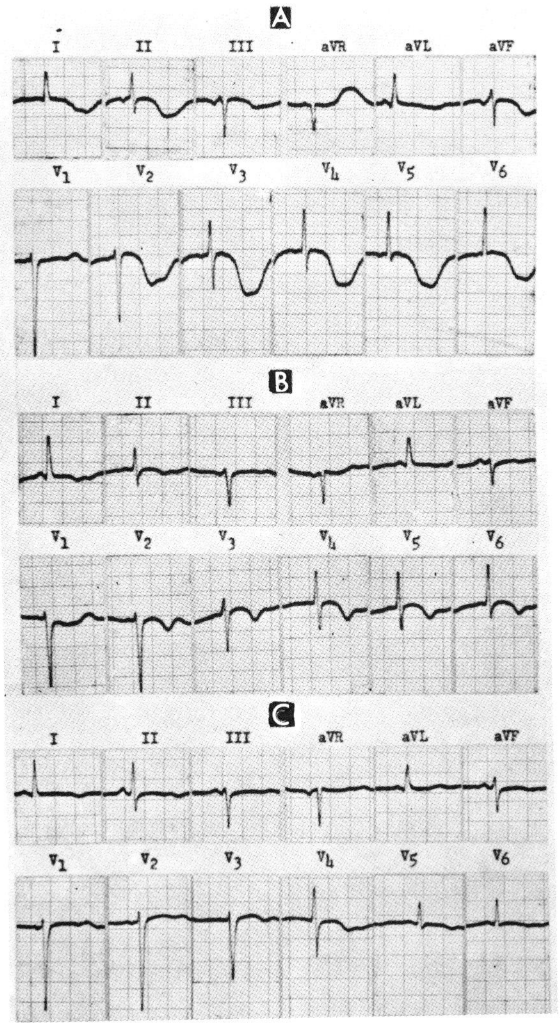

FIG 10–52.
Cerebrovascular accident ECG pattern. 49-year-old woman with a ruptured cerebral aneurysm. **A,** day of admission; observe the wide, bizarre, deeply inverted T waves and prolonged Q-T interval. **B,** 2 days later, note the lessened T wave inversion. **C,** 4 days later, observe further lessening of the T wave inversion. Prominent U waves are present.

11 / Tables

TABLE 1.

QT Interval: Upper Limits of Normal

HEART RATE PER MINUTE	MEN AND CHILDREN (SEC)	WOMEN (SEC)
40	0.49	0.50
45	0.47	0.48
50	0.45	0.46
55	0.43	0.44
60	0.42	0.43
65	0.40	0.42
70	0.39	0.41
75	0.38	0.39
80	0.37	0.38
85	0.36	0.37
90	0.35	0.36
95	0.35	0.36
100	0.34	0.35

TABLE 2.

Rapid Determination of Heart Rate*

DISTANCE BETWEEN 2 QRS COMPLEXES (NO. LARGE SQUARES)	HEART RATE PER MINUTE
1	300
2	150
3	100
4	75
5	60
6	50
7	43
8	37
9	33
10	30

*Simply divide the number of large squares between two consecutive QRS complexes into 300 to determine heart rate.

TABLE 3.

Five-Position Pacemaker Code*

POSITION	I	II	III	IV	V
Category	Chamber(s) paced	Chamber(s) sensed	Mode of response(s)	Programmable functions	Special tachyarrhythmia functions
Letters used	V—Ventricle	V—Ventricle	T—Triggered	P—Programmable (rate and/or output)	B—Bursts
	A—Atrium	A—Atrium	I—Inhibited	M—Multiprogrammable	N—Normal rate N—Completion S—Scanning
	D—Double	D—Double	D—Double† O—None		
		O—None	R—Reverse	O—None	E—External
Manufacturer's designation only	S—Single S—Chamber	S—Single S—Chamber			

*From Lipman BS, Dunn M, Massie E: *Clinical Electrocardiography*, ed 7. Chicago, Year Book Medical Publishers, 1984, p 468. Used by permission.

†Atrial triggered and ventricular inhibited.

TABLE 4.

Treadmill Stress Test—Bruce Protocol*†

AGES (YR)	20	25	30	35	40	45	50	55	60	65	70	75	80
Maximal heart rate (untrained)	197	195	193	191	189	187	184	182	180	178	176	174	172
85% of maximal	167	166	164	162	161	159	156	155	153	151	150	148	146
90% of maximal	177	175	173	172	170	168	166	164	162	160	158	157	155

MULTISTAGE GRADED EXERCISE AT 3-MINUTE INTERVALS

Stage 0	1.0 mph @ 5°
Stage 1	1.7 mph @ 10°
Stage 2	2.5 mph @ 12°
Stage 3	3.4 mph @ 14°
Stage 4	4.2 mph @ 16°
Stage 5	5.0 mph @ 18°

*Adapted from Bruce RA, Rowell LB, Blackman JR, et al: Cardiovascular function tests. *Heart Bull* 1965; 14:9–14. Reproduced with permission from Lipman BS, Dunn M, Massie E: *Clinical Electrocardiography*, ed 7. Chicago, Year Book Medical Publishers, 1984, p 277.

†Target heart rates according to age. Exercise is performed and blood pressure measurements taken and recorded in multistages at 3-minute intervals as the workload is gradually increased. Before exercise, supine, standing, and hyperventilation tracings and blood pressure readings are obtained. After exercise test, recordings and blood pressure readings are obtained at 2-minute, 6-minute, and 10-minute intervals.

Index

B

C

D

E

F

K

L

M

N

O

P

Q

R

S

T

U

V

W